Keto Diet
&
Anti-Inflammatory Diet
- For Beginners -

2 BOOKS IN 1

A Comprehensive Guide to Vibrant Living with Simple, Quick, and Delicious Recipes for Reducing Inflammation and Fortifying the Immune System

Featuring 2 Meal Plans & 2 Exercise Guides

By

Melinda Francis

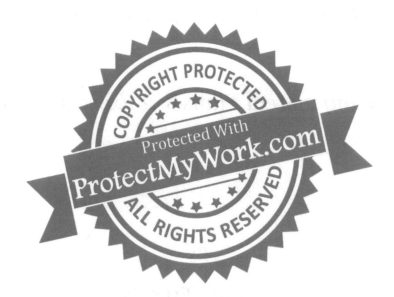

Table of Contents

KETO DIET FOR BEGINNERS

Introduction

The aim of the keto diet is to minimize the intake of carbohydrates to almost negligible levels, triggering the body to utilize fats for energy instead of relying on carbs. This dietary strategy presents two primary advantages: weight management and a potential decrease in the risk of specific ailments. Particularly beneficial for certain demographics, such as young individuals dealing with epilepsy, a high-fat ketogenic diet might offer support. While it isn't a miraculous solution, it stands as one of the available options alongside various antiepileptic medications. For certain individuals, this dietary approach could lead to better seizure control and enhanced cognitive acuity, potentially reducing the dependence on medication. Although adapting to the ketogenic diet might initially appear challenging, with time, familiarity, and a clear comprehension of its goals, it can evolve into a feasible routine. The primary aim of this diet is to substitute carbohydrate sources like sugar and bread with fats as the primary energy source for the body. Achieving this requires a substantial reduction in carb intake, paired with an elevation in the consumption of healthy fats. The diet's strictness demands precise measurement of all food items, accurate to a tenth of a gram during meal preparation. Additionally, participants must exclusively consume foods approved by their dietitian. The carbohydrate limit is so minimal that even the slight sugar content in various liquid or chewable medications could potentially impede the diet's efficacy. For instance, a typical evening meal might include a specific type of meat and leafy vegetables cooked with ample butter or mayonnaise. To sip, heavy cream could be added on the side. Another meal could feature eggs and bacon with a generous amount of oil or butter and heavy cream. For the diet to be effective, an exceptionally high ratio of fats to carbs must be maintained with a low overall calorie intake. A ketogenic diet might serve as an alternative for individuals struggling to shed weight through traditional methods. The optimal ratios of fat, carbs, and protein needed to achieve specific health benefits can vary based on an individual's genetic composition and body structure. Therefore, anyone contemplating the commencement of a ketogenic diet should seek guidance from both their healthcare provider and a registered dietitian. Collaborating with these professionals is vital in devising a personalized meal plan that aligns with their existing health conditions, prevents nutritional deficiencies, and ensures thorough monitoring of any biochemical changes upon embarking on the diet. Furthermore, when reintegrating carbohydrates after a period of weight loss, the expertise of a dietitian can be incredibly valuable in making informed decisions and maintaining a well-rounded nutritional approach.

Chapter 1: Understanding The Ketogenic Diet

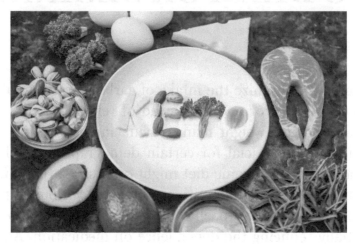

The primary objective of a keto diet is to induce a state of ketosis, wherein the breakdown of body fat produces ketones, enabling the body to predominantly rely on ketones instead of glucose. Various methods can be employed to trigger ketosis, resulting in the existence of multiple variations of the ketogenic diet. Despite the diversity in these approaches, they share common characteristics, primarily emphasizing high dietary fat intake and minimal carbohydrates.

Unveiling Ketosis

A keto diet strives to initiate a metabolic state known as ketosis or a ketogenic state. Ketosis, as a metabolic condition, generates ketone bodies to replace glucose as the primary energy source for the central nervous system and the brain. When carbohydrate intake is insufficient, and the body depletes its glycogen and glucose stores, ketosis is initiated. In the absence of carbohydrates, the body turns to fat for energy, leading to the production of ketones. Typically, ketosis begins a few days into adopting the keto diet. Testing kits are available for assessing ketone levels in urine and blood to confirm the state of ketosis.

Navigating the Keto Flu

The initial two weeks of embarking on the keto diet may present some individuals with what is colloquially known as the "keto flu." Unlike an actual flu, this is a cluster of symptoms resembling flu-like sensations. While the exact cause of the keto flu in some individuals remains unclear, it may be linked to how efficiently one's metabolism adapts to utilizing fat as the primary fuel source instead of carbohydrates.

Potential Symptoms of the Keto Flu Include:

- Headache
- Chills and fever
- Sleep disturbances
- Cravings for sugar
- Fatigue

- Nausea, diarrhea, vomiting, and constipation
- Difficulty concentrating, confusion, and irritability
- Abdominal discomfort

1.1 Varieties Of Ketogenic Diets

Below are the fundamental types of the ketogenic diet.

SKD - Standard Ketogenic Diet. The standard ketogenic diet (SKD) maintains a macronutrient breakdown of approximately 20 percent protein, 70 to 75 percent fat, and around 5 to 10 percent carbohydrates on a daily basis (in grams).

- Protein: 40 to 60g

- Carbohydrates: 20 to 50g

- Unlimited Fat

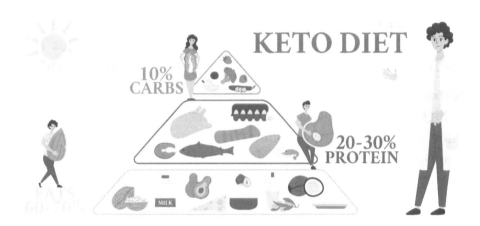

For it to be recognized as a ketogenic diet, fat must constitute the majority of your calorie intake. There is no specific limit as energy requirements can vary widely among individuals. Vegetables, particularly non-starchy ones with minimal carbohydrate content, should play a significant role in ketogenic diets. The Standard Ketogenic Diet (SKD) has consistently demonstrated its effectiveness in aiding weight loss, managing blood sugar levels, and improving cardiovascular health.

WFKD - Well-Formulated Ketogenic Diet. Coined by ketogenic diet pioneer Steve Phinney, the well-formulated ketogenic diet (WFKD) follows a structure similar to the traditional ketogenic diet. It is considered well-formulated when the ratios of protein, macronutrients, fat, and carbohydrates meet, increasing the likelihood of inducing ketosis.

Calorie-restricted ketogenic diet. The only distinction between a regular ketogenic diet and a calorie-restricted one lies in the daily calorie allowance. Research suggests that ketogenic diets can be effective whether or not calorie intake is controlled. This is attributed to the satiating effect of fat consumption in ketosis, aiding in the prevention of overeating.

TKD - Targeted Ketogenic Diet. Despite allowing carbohydrate intake around workouts, the TKD closely resembles the standard ketogenic diet. It serves as a compromise between the strict ketogenic diet and the cyclical one, where carbohydrates can be consumed on workout days. Consuming carbohydrates before or after physical activity is believed to be more readily absorbed by the body due to increased energy demand in active muscles.

VLCKD - Very-low-carb ketogenic diet. Due to its extremely low carb content, a regular ketogenic diet is often referred to as a VLCKD.

Ketogenic Diet MCT. Following the foundational principles of the ketogenic diet, the MCT ketogenic diet emphasizes the use of medium-chain triglycerides (MCTs) as the primary source of dietary fat. MCTs are found in coconut oil, MCT emulsion drinks, and MCT oil. MCT ketogenic diets have been explored in epilepsy treatment, allowing increased protein and carbohydrate intake while maintaining ketosis. It's worth noting that consuming MCTs alone may lead to nausea and diarrhea, and combining them with non-MCT fats in meals is advisable to mitigate these effects. However, research on broader benefits of MCTs for weight loss or blood sugar levels is currently insufficient.

CKD - Cyclical Ketogenic Diet. The CKD diet incorporates days with higher carbohydrate consumption, known as "backloading" days, alternating with days of ketosis (for example, 5 days of ketosis followed by 2 days of increased carbohydrate intake). Athletes are encouraged to leverage the elevated carbohydrate intake on training days to replenish muscle glycogen stores.

High Protein Ketogenic Diet. Distinguished by a higher protein content than the typical ketogenic diet, the high protein ketogenic diet maintains a ratio of 60% fat, 35% protein, and 5% carbohydrates. Some evidence suggests that adhering to a high-protein ketogenic diet may support weight loss. However, there is insufficient information to determine if a long-term high-protein ketogenic diet poses health risks similar to other ketogenic diets.

1.2   Established Benefits Of The Ketogenic Diet

Here are some documented health advantages associated with the keto diet:

- **Enhance cholesterol levels.** The keto diet has demonstrated the ability to positively impact cholesterol levels. Plaque formation and cardiovascular disease, often linked to low-density lipoproteins (LDL) or "bad" cholesterol, can be mitigated by elevating high-density lipoproteins (HDL), known as the "good" cholesterol. Studies have validated that adopting a ketogenic diet can elevate "good" HDL cholesterol levels while reducing levels of "bad" LDL cholesterol, potentially lowering the risk of cardiovascular disease.

- **Improved blood sugar control and insulin resistance.** Effective control of blood sugar and insulin resistance is critical for overall health. The keto diet has shown promise in regulating glucose levels and enhancing insulin sensitivity. Individuals with type 2 diabetes who follow a ketogenic diet may experience improved insulin sensitivity and better blood sugar regulation. It is important for those diagnosed with diabetes and taking medication to consult with their healthcare provider before making significant dietary changes, as medication adjustments may be necessary.

- **Facilitates weight loss.** Weight loss is a widely recognized benefit of the keto diet and a common motivator for its adoption. Numerous studies indicate that the ketogenic diet surpasses low-fat alternatives in achieving rapid, short-term weight loss. While initial weight loss may include a substantial amount of water weight, some research suggests that the keto diet may be particularly effective in reducing abdominal fat, also known as visceral fat. This type of fat, surrounding organs, is associated with an increased risk of chronic conditions like diabetes, fatty liver, and heart disease.

- **Seizure reduction.** The ketogenic diet's historical application for seizure prevention predates the widespread use of anti-seizure medications. Today, it continues to be employed to assist individuals who struggle to control seizures with medication alone.

- **Blood pressure regulation.** Maintaining healthy blood pressure is crucial for preventing conditions such as chronic renal disease, stroke, and heart disease. Research suggests that adopting a ketogenic diet may contribute to lowering blood pressure and promoting cardiovascular health.

Medical Conditions That May See Improvement With A Ketogenic Diet

A ketogenic diet has been suggested as beneficial for various health issues, including:

- **Prediabetes and diabetes.** Insulin resistance is a prevalent feature of prediabetes and type 2 diabetes. Research indicates that the keto diet may enhance insulin sensitivity, potentially aiding in the management of blood sugar levels. Some studies even suggest the potential of the ketogenic diet in addressing type 2 diabetes, potentially reducing the need for diabetic medications.

- **Heart disease.** Individuals at risk of heart-related issues, such as heart attacks, coronary artery disease, and stroke, may find benefits in a ketogenic diet. By addressing risk factors like excessive cholesterol and uncontrolled high blood pressure, the keto diet could contribute to improved heart health.

- **Neurodegenerative diseases.** The state of ketosis induced by the ketogenic diet might have positive implications for neurodegenerative diseases like Parkinson's and Alzheimer's. Preliminary studies propose that a ketogenic diet could alleviate symptoms associated with these conditions. Although the exact mechanisms remain unclear, ketone bodies are believed to play a role in preserving the health of neurons and nerves affected by various neurological illnesses, potentially slowing down the aging process in the brain.

- **Epilepsy.** Phe ketogenic diet has a historical connection with epilepsy treatment, particularly for individuals with seizures that are challenging to control with antiepileptic drugs.

- **Metabolic syndrome.** Conditions encompassed by metabolic syndrome, a cluster of symptoms associated with an increased risk of heart attacks, strokes, and chronic illnesses, may benefit from a ketogenic diet. The five defining conditions of metabolic syndrome include high blood pressure, excess abdominal fat, high cholesterol, elevated blood sugar, and high triglycerides. Some studies suggest that a ketogenic diet may have positive effects on these conditions.

1.3   Contraindications And Risks Of The Ketogenic Diet

Commencing the ketogenic diet poses certain risks, particularly for individuals with specific health conditions:

Diabetes Management Caution. People with diabetes who are on oral hypoglycemic medications or insulin face the risk of severe hypoglycemia if their medications are not carefully adjusted when initiating the ketogenic diet. It is crucial to monitor and adjust medications appropriately to prevent complications.

Medical Conditions Precluding Keto Diet. The ketogenic diet is not recommended for individuals with certain medical conditions, including liver disease, pancreatitis, and disorders related to fat metabolism. Additionally, contraindications encompass carnitine palmitoyl transferase deficiency, primary carnitine deficit, carnitine translocase insufficiency, pyruvate kinase deficiency, and porphyrias. These conditions necessitate careful consideration before embarking on a ketogenic dietary regimen.

False-Positive Alcohol Breath Test. An occasional concern with the ketogenic diet is the potential for a false-positive breath alcohol test result. Ketonemia, a condition associated with the diet, may lead hepatic alcohol dehydrogenase to convert acetone in the body to isopropanol, causing inaccuracies in alcohol breath test outcomes.

Short-Term Adverse Effects. Short-term adverse effects of the ketogenic diet, often referred to as the "keto flu," may include symptoms such as nausea, vomiting, headaches, fatigue, dizziness, and sleep disturbances. These discomforts typically subside within several days to a few weeks. Maintaining proper hydration and replenishing electrolytes can help alleviate these transient symptoms.

Long-Term Ramifications. It is essential to acknowledge potential long-term ramifications of the ketogenic diet, including hepatic steatosis, kidney stones, hypoproteinemia, and the possibility of deficiencies in minerals and vitamins. Monitoring one's health status closely is crucial during prolonged adherence to the ketogenic diet to address and mitigate these potential concerns. Regular health check-ups and consultation with healthcare professionals are advisable for individuals committed to a long-term ketogenic lifestyle.

1.4   Keto Diet Tips: Embrace Keto In 5 Steps

Maximize your success by following these five steps:

1) Define Your Health Objectives

Before embarking on the keto diet, clarify your health goals. What are your intentions? Are you aiming for weight loss or looking to enhance overall health, such as reducing blood sugar levels? Setting clear goals from the outset will keep you motivated and minimize setbacks.

Consider Diabetes Management. For those seeking to lower blood sugar, the keto diet may be an option. Prior to implementation, consult your doctor, especially if using diabetic medication. To prevent hypoglycemia, your doctor may recommend adjusting your diabetic medication dosage.

Regular monitoring of blood sugar levels and potential medication adjustments may be necessary once on a ketogenic diet.

Decide on Ketone Monitoring. Opt to monitor ketone levels to gauge whether you've entered ketosis and adjust your carbohydrate target accordingly. Ketone levels can be measured through breath, urine, or blood tests.

Address High Blood Pressure or Cholesterol. Starting a ketogenic diet may influence blood cholesterol levels, with some individuals experiencing noticeable changes. Consult your doctor to determine if cholesterol levels or other lab tests should be checked post-diet initiation. If on blood pressure medication, discuss potential adjustments, as significant weight loss from any diet may impact blood pressure, necessitating medication modifications.

2) Establish dietary goals

Define your dietary objectives by focusing on protein and carbohydrate targets:

Prioritize Protein Intake. While keto diets provide a moderate amount of protein (around 20% of calories), excessive protein should be avoided to prevent hindrance of ketosis.

High protein intake can lead to glucose production, potentially impeding ketosis.

Set Carb Goals. Choose a percentage or gram goal for carbohydrates, typically ranging from 5 to 10%. Many keto programs start with 20 to 30 grams of "net carbs" daily (total carbs minus fiber). Tracking net carbs allows for increased consumption of nutrient-rich nuts, vegetables, and seeds.

3) Stock Your Kitchen

Transitioning to a ketogenic diet may feel like a significant change, so take time to plan for this new lifestyle. Keep tempting high-carb foods out of your kitchen to stay on track.

Boost your success by stocking your kitchen with keto-friendly foods, including:

- ✔ **Vegetables.** Leafy greens like spinach, kale, and lettuce, as well as low-carb options like asparagus, broccoli, bell peppers, zucchini, and cauliflower.
- ✔ **Protein-Rich Meats and Foods.** Opt for fresh meats, fish, poultry, tofu, chicken, turkey, pork, beef, and eggs over processed meats.
- ✔ **Dairy and substitutes.** Allowable options include cheese, sour cream, butter, coconut milk, cream, and unsweetened almond milk.
- ✔ **Seasonings & Spices.** Most herbs and spices are acceptable in moderation.
- ✔ **Oils and Fats.** Embrace healthy options like flaxseed, avocado, olive, and walnut oils.
- ✔ **Fruit.** Limited options like lemon, blueberries, raspberries, tomatoes, and avocados are permitted.
- ✔ **Seeds and Nuts.** Enjoyed in moderation as sources of beneficial minerals and healthy fats.
- ✔ **Beverages.** Include coffee, sparkling water, broth, tea, and water.

4) Enhance Dietary Intake

Optimize your keto diet experience by:

Choosing Healthy Fats. Ensure adequate consumption of healthy fats such as avocados, olive oil, avocado oil, seeds, and nuts, alongside sausage and cream.

Developing a Fiber Strategy. Given the limitations on fiber-containing carbs, maximize vegetable intake while staying within your net carb limit. Consider incorporating low-carb fiber sources like chia seeds and flax seeds or, if needed, explore fiber supplements.

Increasing Hydration and Salt Intake. Fluid losses may rise on a keto diet, particularly in the initial weeks. Maintain hydration by keeping a water bottle nearby and consuming carb-free beverages. Adjust salt intake if needed, especially in the early weeks to prevent symptoms like headaches and dizziness associated with the "keto flu."

Supplementing with Minerals or Multivitamins. Certain vitamins and minerals like B vitamins, calcium, magnesium, and potassium may be insufficient in a keto diet, even with careful planning. Consider supplementing with minerals or multivitamins, ensuring they align with the low-carb nature of your diet.

5) Seek Support

Inform your support network about your goals and enlist their help. Having a supportive community can significantly impact your chances of success. Share your objectives and let your loved ones know how they can contribute to your journey.

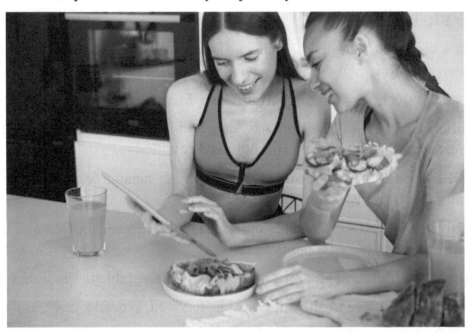

Chapter 2: Shopping Guide - KETO GROCERY LIST

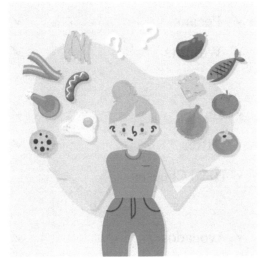

Here's a comprehensive shopping list to guide your keto shopping spree:

Foods to Include

Here's a comprehensive shopping list to guide your keto shopping spree:

Vegetables

✓ Asparagus	✓ Radishes	✓ Kale
✓ Brussels Sprouts	✓ Spinach	✓ Mushrooms
✓ Cauliflower	✓ Zucchini	✓ Onion
✓ Cucumber	✓ Artichokes	✓ Pumpkin
✓ Green Beans	✓ Broccoli	✓ Sauerkraut
✓ Lettuce	✓ Cabbage	✓ Tomatoes
✓ Okra	✓ Celery	
✓ Peppers	✓ Garlic	

Meats

✓ Ground Beef	✓ Smoked Deli Meats	✓ Beef Jerky
✓ Chicken (all cuts)	✓ Fish & Shellfish	✓ Ham
✓ Pork	✓ Bacon	✓ Pepperoni
✓ Duck	✓ Beef	✓ Hotdogs
✓ Sausages	✓ Turkey	
✓ Pastrami	✓ Wild Game	

Seeds & Nuts

- ✓ Almonds
- ✓ Macadamias
- ✓ Sunflower Seeds
- ✓ Flaxseeds
- ✓ Pecans
- ✓ Walnuts
- ✓ Peanuts (your choice)
- ✓ Chia Seeds
- ✓ Pumpkin Seeds

Dairy

- ✓ Heavy Cream
- ✓ Soft Cheeses
- ✓ Cottage Cheese
- ✓ Mayo
- ✓ Butter
- ✓ Hard Cheeses
- ✓ Sour Cream
- ✓ Greek Yogurt (low-carb)

Fruits

- ✓ Berries
- ✓ Lime
- ✓ Avocados
- ✓ Lemon
- ✓ Coconut (unsweetened)

Fats

- ✓ Coconut Oil
- ✓ MCT Oil
- ✓ Lard
- ✓ Cocoa Butter
- ✓ Avocado Oil
- ✓ Olive Oil
- ✓ Ghee
- ✓ Bacon Fat

Flour & Eggs

- ✓ Almond
- ✓ Coconut
- ✓ Psyllium Husk
- ✓ Eggs

Pantry Items

- ✓ Chicken Broth
- ✓ Bone Broth
- ✓ Pork Rinds
- ✓ Beef Broth
- ✓ Xanthan Gum
- ✓ Tabasco
- ✓ Coconut or Braggs Amino
- ✓ Herbs & Spices
- ✓ Salad Dressings (low-carb)
- ✓ Baking Cocoa Powder
- ✓ Sweeteners
- ✓ Parchment Paper
- ✓ Pickles

Nut Butter Unsweetened

- ✓ Macadamia Nut Butter
- ✓ Peanut Butter (any of your choice)
- ✓ Almond Butter
- ✓ Coconut Butter

Foods to Avoid

Grains

- Oatmeal
- Quinoa
- Corn
- Flour & corn tortillas
- Barley
- Sandwich wraps
- Rye
- Pumpernickel
- Sorghum
- Oats
- WhiteWheat
- Rice
- Buckwheat
- Sourdough

Legumes

- Chickpeas
- Cannellini beans
- Black beans
- Pinto beans
- Navy beans
- Lentils
- Black-eyed peas
- Baked beans
- Kidney beans
- Green peas
- Lima beans
- Great Northern beans

Fruit

- Oranges
- Nectarines
- Grapes
- Bananas
- Tangerines
- Mangos
- Pears
- Pineapples
- Peaches
- Fruit Juices
- Apples
- Fruit smoothies
- Dried fruits such as dates, raisins, and dried mango
- All fruit juices (excluding lime juice and lemon)

Dairy

- Condensed milk
- Most kinds of milk
- Low-fat or fat-free yogurt
- Creamed cottage cheese

Vegetables

- Sweet potatoes
- Parsnips
- Peas
- Yams
- Potatoes
- Artichoke
- Corn
- Baked potatoes
- Cassava (Yuca)

Protein

× Breaded meats

× Bacon with added sugar

× Other processed meats that might have hidden carbs

Beverages

× Hot Chocolate

× Grape Soda

× Tonic Water (Not sugar-free)

× Sports Drinks

× Fruit juices

× Sweetened iced tea

× Mocha

× Colas

× Ginger Ale

× Root Beer

× Energy Drinks (Not sugar-free)

× Vitamin Water

× Lemonade

× Frappuccino

× Non-light beers

× Cocktails like screwdrivers, margaritas, and piña coladas

Oils and Other Unhealthy Fats

Ensure a sufficient intake of fats in your keto diet, including recommended additional fats like oils (2 to 4 teaspoons per day).

Chapter 3: Keto And Exercise

Before you venture into the combination of the ketogenic diet and physical activity, there are several crucial factors that experts highlight. The ketogenic diet, commonly known as keto, has gained considerable popularity, especially among fitness enthusiasts. However, being well-informed about specific critical aspects is essential if you plan to engage in physical activity while adhering to this dietary approach. While the keto diet may provide performance benefits, there are potential challenges to be mindful of, especially during the initial stages of adaptation. Ramsey Bergeron, a keto athlete and NASM-certified personal trainer, warns that the initial days on a keto diet may bring about a feeling of mental fog. This is a result of the body's transition from using glucose (derived from carbohydrates) as its primary energy source to utilizing ketone bodies produced from the breakdown of fats. This transitional period can impact cognitive clarity and overall well-being. Bergeron suggests avoiding activities that demand rapid reactions, such as biking in traffic, during this phase.

Incorporating Exercise and the Ketogenic Diet

✓ **Gradual Transition:** It is advisable to ease into the ketogenic diet rather than making sudden changes. Abrupt carbohydrate restriction may cause discomfort and hinder exercise performance.

✓ **Adequate Fuel:** Consuming sufficient energy before exercising is crucial, as the ketogenic diet may inadvertently lead to undereating. The appetite-suppressing effects of ketosis might mask the body's need for fuel, potentially affecting workout performance.

✓ **Low-Intensity Workouts:** The ketogenic diet's impact on utilizing ketone bodies and fat for energy can enhance fat oxidation and spare glycogen during low- to moderate-intensity aerobic exercises like running or biking. While high-intensity performance may be compromised due to reduced glycogen stores, moderate exercise can still be effective for fat burning.

✓ **High-Intensity Exercises:** Activities requiring bursts of high-intensity effort, like CrossFit or HIIT, may not align well with the ketogenic diet due to glycogen depletion. Consider adopting the ketogenic diet during off-season periods or when performance optimization is not the primary goal.

✓ **Sufficient Fat Intake:** Adequate fat consumption is essential to prevent negative outcomes and optimize exercise benefits while on a ketogenic diet. Falling short on fat intake can lead to hunger, muscle loss, and hindered ketosis. Opt for healthy fat sources like fish, grass-fed meats, coconut oil, and avocado.

✓ **Listen to Your Body:** Pay close attention to your body's signals, particularly in the initial weeks of combining keto with exercise. If you experience persistent fatigue, lightheadedness, or exhaustion, your body might not be adapting well to a very low-carb diet. Prioritize your overall health and well-being, and consider adjusting your carbohydrate intake if needed.

Integrating the ketogenic diet with exercise requires a nuanced approach that aligns with your individual goals and your body's response.

While the keto diet can potentially enhance fat oxidation and provide energy for certain exercise intensities, careful consideration of nutrient intake and overall well-being is paramount. As you embark on this journey, remember that your body's response may vary, and it's essential to prioritize long-term health and sustainable practices.

3.1 14-Day Fitness Program For Women

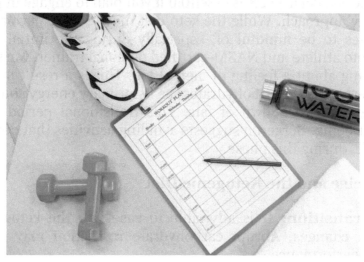

Week 1: Embarking on the Journey

Day 1:
- ✓ Morning: 15-minute brisk walk
- ✓ Afternoon: 10 minutes of bodyweight squats (Instructions: Stand with feet shoulder-width apart, lower into a squat position, then rise back up) and 10 minutes of plank holds (Instructions: Maintain a straight line from head to heels while propped on forearms)
- ✓ Evening: 20 minutes of serene yoga focusing on flexibility (Instructions: Flow through gentle poses, emphasizing deep stretches)

Day 2:
- ✓ Morning: 15-minute brisk walk
- ✓ Afternoon: 20 minutes of utilizing resistance bands for arms (Instructions: Perform bicep curls, lateral raises, and tricep extensions) and legs (Instructions: Incorporate squats, side leg lifts, and leg curls)
- ✓ Evening: 15-minute session of meditation for relaxation (Instructions: Find a quiet space, sit comfortably, focus on your breath, and let go of tension)

Day 3:
- ✓ Morning: 20 minutes of bodyweight lunges (Instructions: Step forward with one foot, lower your hips, and alternate legs) and performing push-ups (Instructions: Maintain a straight body, lower and lift using arms)
- ✓ Afternoon: 10 minutes of low-impact aerobics (e.g., dancing or swimming)
- ✓ Evening: 15 minutes of profound stretching and engaging in yoga poses (Instructions: Include poses like Downward Dog, Cobra, and Child's Pose)

Day 4:
Rest day: Concentrate on staying active with gentle activities like walking or stretching

Day 5:
- ✓ <u>Morning:</u> 20 minutes of high-intensity interval training (HIIT) (Instructions: Alternating short bursts of intense exercises with brief rest periods)
- ✓ <u>Afternoon:</u> 10 minutes of exercises to strengthen the core (Instructions: Plank variations, crunches, and leg raises)
- ✓ <u>Evening:</u> 15 minutes of meditation to alleviate stress (Instructions: Similar to Day 2)

Day 6:
- ✓ <u>Morning:</u> 15-minute brisk walk
- ✓ <u>Afternoon:</u> 20 minutes of yoga to enhance strength and balance (Instructions: Focus on poses that challenge balance, such as Tree Pose and Warrior poses)
- ✓ <u>Evening:</u> 10 minutes of using a foam roller for muscle recovery (Instructions: Roll over targeted muscle groups to release tension)

Day 7:
- ✓ <u>Morning:</u> 15-minute brisk walk
- ✓ <u>Afternoon:</u> 20 minutes of resistance band exercises for a full-body workout (Instructions: Incorporate various exercises targeting different muscle groups)
- ✓ <u>Evening:</u> 15 minutes of deep stretching and relaxation (Instructions: Emphasize full-body stretches, holding each position)

Week 2: Building Momentum

Day 8:
- ✓ <u>Morning:</u> 20 minutes of bodyweight squats and lunges (Instructions: Perform squats and lunges, ensuring proper form and controlled movements)
- ✓ <u>Afternoon:</u> 15 minutes of low-impact aerobics (Instructions: Engage in activities like brisk walking, step-ups, and side leg lifts)
- ✓ <u>Evening:</u> 10 minutes of mindfulness meditation (Instructions: Find a quiet space, focus on your breath, and cultivate present awareness)

Day 9:
- ✓ <u>Morning:</u> 20 minutes of High-Intensity Interval Training (HIIT) (Instructions: Incorporate exercises like jumping jacks, burpees, and mountain climbers in short bursts)
- ✓ <u>Afternoon:</u> 10 minutes of core strengthening exercises (Instructions: Include exercises like planks, Russian twists, and leg raises)
- ✓ <u>Evening:</u> 15 minutes of yoga for flexibility (Instructions: Emphasize poses like Cobra, Downward Dog, and Seated Forward Bend)

Day 10:
<u>Rest day:</u> Engage in light activities like walking or gentle stretching

Day 11:
- ✓ <u>Morning:</u> 15-minute brisk walk
- ✓ <u>Afternoon:</u> 20 minutes of resistance band exercises for arms and legs (Instructions: Use resistance bands for bicep curls, leg presses, and lateral raises)
- ✓ <u>Evening:</u> 10 minutes of foam rolling for muscle recovery (Instructions: Roll over targeted muscle groups to release tension)

Day 12:
- ✓ <u>Morning:</u> 20 minutes of yoga for strength and balance (Instructions: Focus on poses that challenge balance, such as Warrior poses and Tree Pose)
- ✓ <u>Afternoon:</u> 15 minutes of low-impact aerobics (Instructions: Include activities like dancing or swimming with controlled movements)
- ✓ <u>Evening:</u> 15 minutes of meditation for relaxation (Instructions: Similar to previous meditation sessions)

Day 13:
- ✓ <u>Morning:</u> 15-minute brisk
- ✓ <u>Afternoon:</u> 20 minutes of bodyweight exercises for the whole body (Instructions: Perform exercises like squats, push-ups, and lunges
- ✓ <u>Evening:</u> 10 minutes of deep stretching and stress relief (Instructions: Emphasize full-body stretches, holding each position)

Day 14:
- ✓ <u>Morning:</u> 20 minutes of HIIT
- ✓ <u>Afternoon:</u> 10 minutes of core strengthening exercises
- ✓ <u>Evening:</u> 15 minutes of mindfulness meditation

Tips:
- Maintain hydration throughout the day.
- Ensure your dietary choices align with your ketogenic and anti-inflammatory objectives.
- Pay attention to your body, and if you experience excessive fatigue or discomfort, adjust the exercises accordingly.
- If you have preexisting health concerns, it is recommended that you consult with a doctor before initiating an exercise regimen.

3.2 14-Day Exercise Plan For Men

Week 1: Commencing the Journey

Day 1:
- ✓ <u>Morning:</u> 20-minute brisk
- ✓ <u>Afternoon:</u> 15 minutes of bodyweight squats and push-ups (Instructions: Perform squats with proper form, followed by push-ups targeting chest and triceps
- ✓ <u>Evening:</u> 20 minutes of gentle yoga for flexibility (Instructions: Focus on stretches that enhance overall flexibility)

Day 2:
- ✓ <u>Morning:</u> 20-minute brisk walk
- ✓ <u>Afternoon:</u> 20 minutes of resistance band exercises for full-body strength (Instructions: Utilize resistance bands for exercises like bicep curls, leg presses, and lateral raises)
- ✓ <u>Evening:</u> 15 minutes of meditation for relaxation (Instructions: Find a quiet space, concentrate on breathing, and cultivate a state of relaxation)

Day 3:
- ✓ <u>Morning:</u> 25 minutes of bodyweight lunges and planking (Instructions: Perform lunges with controlled movements and engage in planks for core strength)
- ✓ <u>Afternoon:</u> 15 minutes of low-impact aerobics (e.g., cycling or swimming)
- ✓ <u>Evening:</u> 20 minutes of deep stretching and yoga (Instructions: Emphasize yoga poses that promote flexibility and muscle relaxation)

Day 4:
<u>Rest day:</u> Focus on staying active with light activities such as walking or stretching

Day 5:
- ✓ <u>Morning:</u> 25 minutes of high-intensity interval training (HIIT) (Instructions: Include exercises like jumping jacks, burpees, and mountain climbers in short, intense bursts)
- ✓ <u>Afternoon:</u> 15 minutes of core strengthening exercises (Instructions: Incorporate exercises like planks, Russian twists, and leg raises)
- ✓ <u>Evening:</u> 20 minutes of mindfulness meditation (Instructions: Similar to previous meditation sessions)

Day 6:
- ✓ <u>Morning:</u> 20-minute brisk walk
- ✓ <u>Afternoon:</u> 25 minutes of yoga for strength and balance (Instructions: Focus on poses that challenge balance, such as Warrior poses and Tree Pose)
- ✓ <u>Evening:</u> 15 minutes of foam rolling for muscle recovery (Instructions: Use a foam roller to target muscle groups and release tension)

Day 7:
- ✓ <u>Morning:</u> 20-minute brisk walk
- ✓ <u>Afternoon:</u> 25 minutes of resistance band exercises for arms and legs (Instructions: Engage in a full-body workout using resistance bands)
- ✓ <u>Evening:</u> 20 minutes of deep stretching and relaxation (Instructions: Incorporate stretches that promote relaxation and alleviate muscle tension)

Week 2: Igniting Momentum

Day 8:
- ✓ <u>Morning:</u> Engage in a 25-minute session of bodyweight squats and lunges (Instructions: Execute squats and lunges with proper form, focusing on controlled movements and engaging leg muscles
- ✓ <u>Afternoon:</u> Embrace a 20-minute low-impact aerobics session (Instructions: Include activities like walking or cycling with reduced joint impact
- ✓ <u>Evening:</u> Dedicate 15 minutes to mindfulness meditation (Instructions: Find a quiet space, focus on your breath, and cultivate a state of mindful awareness)

Day 9:
- ✓ <u>Morning:</u> Invest 25 minutes in a High-Intensity Interval Training (HIIT) session (Instructions: Perform intervals of intense exercises followed by short rest periods for a challenging workout)
- ✓ <u>Afternoon:</u> Devote 15 minutes to core strengthening exercises (Instructions: Include exercises like planks, crunches, and leg raises)

✓ Evening: Engage in a 20-minute yoga session emphasizing flexibility (Instructions: Incorporate yoga poses that enhance flexibility and stretching)

Day 10:
Rest day: Participate in light activities such as walking or gentle stretching to promote recovery and relaxation

Day 11:
- ✓ Morning: Embark on a 20-minute brisk walk to invigorate the body
- ✓ Afternoon: Dedicate 25 minutes to resistance band exercises for a full-body workout (Instructions: Utilize resistance bands for various exercises targeting different muscle groups)
- ✓ Evening: Allocate 15 minutes for foam rolling to aid muscle recovery (Instructions: Use a foam roller to target specific muscle groups and alleviate muscle tension)

Day 12:
- ✓ Morning: Immerse yourself in a 25-minute yoga session focusing on strength and balance (Instructions: Include yoga poses that challenge balance and promote overall strength)
- ✓ Afternoon: Embrace a 20-minute low-impact aerobics session
- ✓ Evening: Engage in a 20-minute meditation for relaxation and mental rejuvenation

Day 13:
- ✓ Morning: Participate in a 20-minute brisk walk to stimulate the body
- ✓ Afternoon: Invest 25 minutes in bodyweight exercises for the entire body (Instructions: Include exercises like push-ups, squats, and lunges)
- ✓ Evening: Dedicate 15 minutes to deep stretching and stress relief

Day 14:
- ✓ Morning: Commit to a 25-minute HIIT session for an intense workout experience
- ✓ Afternoon: Devote 15 minutes to core strengthening exercises
- ✓ Evening: Engage in a 20-minute mindfulness meditation session

Tips:
- Ensure you stay well-hydrated throughout the day.
- Align your diet with your ketogenic and anti-inflammatory goals for optimal results.
- Pay careful attention to your body and adapt exercises as needed, particularly if you experience extreme fatigue or discomfort.
- If you have preexisting health conditions, consult with your doctor before commencing a new exercise routine.

Chapter 4: Appetizers, Snacks & Side Dishes Recipes

Below are the recipes.

1. Rosemary Toasted Nuts

(Setup Time: 5 minutes | Cooked in: 10 minutes | How many people 5 | Difficulty: Easy)

Recipe Components:

- 2 tsps fresh rosemary leaves, finely chopped
- 1 tsp erythritol
- ⅛ tsp black pepper, ground
- 200 g or 1¼ cups raw almonds
- 2 tbsp coconut oil or ghee
- 1¼ tsps sea salt, finely ground
- ½ tsp cumin, ground
- Pinch of cayenne pepper

Preparation Steps: Melt the oil in a large frying pan over low heat. Cayenne, cumin, salt, erythritol, and rosemary should be mixed in after the butter has melted. As you mix, sprinkle on the almonds. For 5–8 minutes, or until a light brown color develops, cook the almonds while stirring them every 30 seconds. Take the food off the heat and let it cool fully before eating.

Nutritional Info: Calories: 300 kcal, Protein: 8.5g, Carb: 9g, Fat: 25.6g.

2. Mushroom Breaded Nuggets

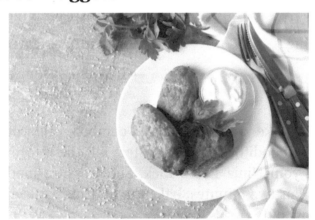

(Setup Time: 15 minutes | Cooked in: 50 minutes | How many people 4 | Difficulty: Easy)

Recipe Components:

- 2 eggs, large
- 1 tsp garlic powder
- ½ tsp sea salt, finely ground
- 120 ml or ½ cup honey mustard dressing, to serve (optional)
- 455 g or 1 lb. about 24 cremini mushrooms

- 55 g or ½ cup blanched almond flour
- 1 tsp paprika
- 2 tbsp avocado oil
- Toothpicks (optional)

Preparation Steps: Set the oven to 177 degrees C (350 F). Line a rimmed baking sheet with a silicone baking mat or parchment paper. Break or trim the mushroom stems so that they are the same height as the caps. In a small dish, break the eggs and give them a good whisk. Sift the almond flour, paprika, garlic powder, and salt into a medium bowl and whisk to combine. Dip the mushrooms one at a time into the eggs, then gently place them into the flour mixture without getting any flour on your hands. To ensure that the mushrooms are evenly coated on all sides, use a fork to toss them in the flour mixture before transferring them to the prepared baking sheet. Apply the same method to the remaining mushrooms. The mushrooms on the cover should be drizzled with oil. About 50 minutes in the oven should be enough time for the tops to brown. Take them out of the oven and serve them with the dressing if you like. Make sure your guests and family members have toothpicks if you have that many.

Nutritional Info: Calories: 332 kcal, Protein: 8g, Carb: 9.3g, Fat: 29.3g.

3. Vanilla muffins

(Setup Time: 5 minutes | Cooked in: 2 minutes | How many people 4 | Difficulty: Easy)

Recipe Components:

- 1 beaten egg
- 1 cup water for cooking
- 1 tsp. vanilla extract
- 1 tbsp. Truvia
- 4 tbsp. coconut flour
- 1 tsp. coconut shred
- ¼ tsp. baking powder

Preparation Steps: To make a thick batter, combine all your ingredients and whisk thoroughly. Inside the Ninja Foodi basket, add water. Fill the muffin tins with the batter, and then place the muffins on your Ninja Foodi rack. Set Pressure mode and lower the pressure cooker's cover. High stress For two minutes, bake the muffins. Utilize the rapid pressure release technique. Serve the muffins cold.

Nutritional Info: Calories: 61 kcal, Protein: 2.5g, Carb: 7g, Fat: 2.9g.

4. Liver Bites

(Setup Time: 10 minutes + 24 hours (soaking time) | Cooked in: 28 minutes | How many people 24 | Difficulty: Hard)

Recipe Components:

- 1 tbsp. apple cider vinegar
- 455 g or 1 pound beef, ground

- 12 cloves garlic, minced
- 1 tsp black pepper, ground
- ½ tsp sea salt, finely ground
- 225 g or 8 ozs of chicken livers
- 4½ oz. or 4 strips of bacon
- 75 g or 1 cup pork rinds, crushed
- 1 tbsp. + 1 tsp onion powder
- 1 tsp thyme leaves, dried

Preparation Steps: Chicken livers should be placed in a medium-sized dish and covered with water. Put vinegar in it. Keep refrigerated for up to 2 days if covered. After washing, the livers should be drained. Set the oven temperature to 190 degrees C (375 F). Line a rimmed baking sheet with a silicone baking mat or parchment paper.

Use a high-powered blender to puree the livers and bacon until there are no chunks left. Chop the bacon first if using a regular food processor or blender. The remaining ingredients can be added to the liver mixture after it has been transferred to a medium bowl. Use your hands to thoroughly combine the items. Pinch and roll a heaping spoonful of the mixture between your palms before placing it on a baking sheet lined with parchment paper. Roll the remaining liver mixture into another 24 balls and repeat the process. Bake the liver balls for 25 to 28 minutes or until the center registers 165 degrees Fahrenheit (74 degrees Celsius).

Nutritional Info: Calories: 116 kcal, Protein: 11.4g, Carb: 1.1g, Fat: 7.4g.

5. Jicama Crunchy Fries

(Setup Time: 5 minutes | Cooked in: 40 minutes | How many people 4 | Difficulty: Easy)

Recipe Components:

- 2 tbsp avocado oil
- 1 pinch of sea salt, finely ground
- 1 lb. or 1 medium jicama, peeled and chopped into fry-like pieces
- ½ tsp paprika
- 1 tsp fresh parsley, finely chopped

Optional (for serving):

- Sugar-free ketchup
- 105 g or ½ cup mayonnaise

Preparation Steps: Prepare a hot oven, preferably at 205 degrees C (400 F). Line a rimmed baking sheet with a silicone baking mat or parchment paper. Jicama pieces should be placed on a baking pan and mixed with paprika and oil. Fries should be baked for 40 minutes, turning them over halfway through. After taking the fries out of the oven, season them with parsley and salt, then serve. If preferred, provide the mayonnaise over the side for dipping.

Nutritional Info: Calories: 96 kcal, Protein: 1.2g, Carb: 14.7g, Fat: 3.7g.

6. Almond bites

(Setup Time: 10 minutes | Cooked in: 14 minutes | How many people 5 | Difficulty: Easy)

Recipe Components:

- ¼ cup almond milk
- 2 tbsp. Butter
- ½ tsp. baking powder
- ½ tsp. vanilla extract
- 1 cup almond flour
- 1 egg, whisked
- 1 tbsp. coconut flakes
- ½ tsp. apple cider vinegar

Preparation Steps: The beaten egg, apple cider vinegar, almond milk, baking powder, butter, and vanilla extract should all be combined. Add coconut flakes and almond flour after stirring the mixture. Work the dough. Almond flour should be added extra once the dough is sticky. Roll the dough into even balls and place them on the rack. Gently press them with the palm of your hand. Cook them all for about 12 minutes at 360 degrees Fahrenheit with the cover of the air fryer. Verify the bite's readiness and cook for 2 minutes for a crispy crust.

Nutritional Info: Calories: 118 kcal, Protein: 2.7g, Carb: 2.4g, Fat: 11.5g.

7. Tuna Cucumber Boats

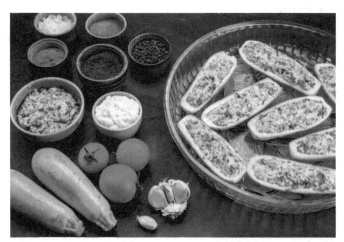

(Setup Time: 5 minutes | Cooked in: 0 minutes | How many people 1 | Difficulty: Easy)

Recipe Components:

- 5-oz/142-g 1 can flake tuna packed inside water, drained
- 3 tbsp mayonnaise
- 2 tsps fresh parsley, finely chopped
- 1 minced clove garlic
- 12 inches/ 30.5 cm long 1 English cucumber
- 1 finely diced dill pickle
- 2 tbsp red onions, finely diced

- 1 tsp lemon juice
- ½ tsp Dijon mustard

Preparation Steps: Using a sharp knife, halve the cucumber lengthwise. Get rid of and store the seeds. Combine the rest of the ingredients in a medium bowl and stir until uniform. Fill each cucumber half with the tuna salad mixture. Place on a dish, and then eat!

Nutritional Info: Calories: 527 kcal, Protein: 41.7g, Carb: 12.7g, Fat: 34.4g.

8. Tapenade

(Setup Time: 5 minutes | Cooked in: 0 minutes | How many people 6 | Difficulty: Easy)

Recipe Components:

- 115 g or 1 cup pitted green olives
- 6 basil leaves, fresh
- 1 tbsp. parsley leaves, fresh
- Leaves from 1 sprig of fresh oregano
- 1 anchovy fillet
- 6 medium celery stalks, cut into sticks to serve
- 115 g or 1 cup pitted black olives
- 28 g or ¼ cup tomatoes in oil, sun-dried and drained
- 1 tbsp. capers
- 2 tsps thyme leaves, fresh
- 1 clove garlic
- 60 ml or ¼ cup olive oil

Preparation Steps: Blend everything element (except the celery and olive oil) until smooth. Pulse it until it's roughly chopped. Once you've added the olive oil, pulse again to combine. Serve in a bowl, and surround it with celery sticks to serve.

Nutritional Info: Calories: 167 kcal, Protein: 0.9g, Carb: 4.1g, Fat: 16.4g.

9. Vanilla Yogurt

(Setup Time: 20 minutes | Cooked in: 3 hours | How many people 4 | Difficulty: Easy)

Recipe Components:

- ¼ cup yogurt started
- ½ tbsp. pure vanilla extract
- ½ cup milk, full-fat
- 1 cup heavy cream
- 2 tsps stevia

Preparation Steps: In the Ninja Foodi pot, combine the milk with the heavy cream, vanilla essence, and Stevia. Sit the yogurt down and secure the cover. 3 hours of cooking in the slow cooker. Mix 1 cup milk and the yogurt starter in a small basin, then pour the mixture into the cooker. Lock the lid and cover the Foodi with two little T-clothes. 9 hours should pass to enable the yogurt to ferment. Serve after refrigeration. Enjoy!

Nutritional Info: Calories: 292 kcal, Protein: 5g, Carb: 8g, Fat: 26g.

10.   Sautéed Asparagus along Tahini-Lemon Sauce

(Setup Time: 5 minutes | Cooked in: 10 minutes | How many people 4 | Difficulty: Easy)

Recipe Components:

- 2 tbsp avocado oil
- 16 asparagus spears, snapped off woody ends

Tahini-Lemon Sauce:

- 1 tbsp. avocado oil
- 1 clove garlic, small minced
- 1 pinch of black pepper, ground
- 2 tbsp tahini
- 2½ tsps lemon juice
- 1/16 tsp sea salt, finely ground
- 1 to 1½ tbsp water

Preparation Steps: Put the oil and asparagus in a large frying pan and heat it over medium heat. Cook for about 10 minutes, occasionally tossing the spears in the oil. Cook over medium heat until they are a light brown color. In the meantime, prepare the sauce. To make the dressing, whisk together 1 tbsp. of water, oil, tahini, lemon juice, salt, garlic, and pepper. Blend until combined. Add the extra 1/2 tbsp of water, and then whisk the dressing once more if it is too thick. Arrange the cooked asparagus and top with the lemon-tahini sauce on a serving platter.

Nutritional Info: Calories: 106 kcal, Protein: 3.5g, Carb: 5.7g, Fat: 7.7g.

11.   Avocado bacon-wrapped fries

(Setup Time: 10 minutes | Cooked in: 18 minutes | How many people 4 | Difficulty: Easy)

Recipe Components:

- 2 medium Hass avocados, pitted and peeled (around 8 oz./220 g of flesh)
- 1 lb./455 g 16 strips bacon, cut in half lengthwise

Preparation Steps: For a total of 16 fries, cut every avocado into 8 pieces in the form of fries. Each avocado fry is encased in two bacon half-strips. Once finished, put it inside a big frying pan.

Cover the pan with a splash protector and heat it over a moderate flame. Cook in oil at 350 degrees for 12 minutes (6 minutes on each side and 6 minutes on the bottom). Take the food out of the heat right away and enjoy!

Nutritional Info: Calories: 525 kcal, Protein: 43.2g, Carb: 6.4g, Fat: 58.3g.

12.   MAC Fatties

(Setup Time: 10 minutes | Cooked in: 0 minutes | How many people 20 | Difficulty: Hard)

Recipe Components:

- 70 g or ⅓ cup coconut oil
- 280 g or 1¾ cups macadamia nuts, salted and roasted

Spicy Cumin Flavor:

- ¼ tsp cayenne pepper
- ½ tsp cumin, ground

Garlic Herb Flavor:

- ½ tsp paprika
- 1¼ tsps oregano leaves, dried
- ½ tsp garlic powder

Rosemary Lemon Flavor:

- ¼ tsp lemon juice
- 1 tsp fresh rosemary, finely chopped

Turmeric Flavor:

- ¼ tsp ginger powder
- ½ tsp turmeric powder

Preparation Steps: Oil and macadamia nuts should be blended or processed together. To the extent that your blender will allow, blend the ingredients until they are entirely smooth. Each of the four little dishes needs a quarter cup (87 g) of the ingredients. Combine the lemon juice and rosemary in the first bowl. Add the cumin and cayenne pepper to a separate bowl and stir to combine. Incorporate the ginger and turmeric into the third bowl. In a separate dish, combine the paprika, oregano, and garlic powder with a whisk. Put a tiny muffin tin or a silicone pan with 24 wells on the counter. Insert tiny foil liners into 20 wells if using a metal pan. (Don't use paper since it will soak up all the grease.) When placing the mixtures in the wells, use about a tbsp. of each combination. Please put it in the freezer for at least an hour or until it's frozen solid. Have it cold, straight from the freezer.

Nutritional Info: Calories: 139 kcal, Protein: 1.1g, Carb: 1.9g, Fat: 14.1g.

13.   Keto Diet Snack Plate

(Setup Time: 10 minutes | Cooked in: 10 minutes | How many people 1 | Difficulty: Easy)

Recipe Components:

- 6 jalapeño-stuffed olives
- 1 medium Hass avocado, pitted, peeled, and sliced (around 4 oz./110 g of flesh)
- 1 tbsp. mayonnaise
- 85 g or 3 ozs salami, sliced
- 28 g or ¼ cup sauerkraut
- 1 large egg, hard-boiled, cut in half, and peeled
- 0.35-oz/10-g 1 package seaweed sheets, roasted

Preparation Steps: Put everything on a dish, and then start eating!

Nutritional Info: Calories: 519 kcal, Protein: 19.7g, Carb: 14.9g, Fat: 57.7g.

14.   Dried tomatoes

(Setup Time: 5 minutes | Cooked in: 8 hours | How many people 8 | Difficulty: Easy)

Recipe Components:

- 1 tbsp. basil
- 1 tbsp. onion powder
- 1 tsp paprika
- 5 tomatoes, medium
- 1 tsp cilantro
- 5 tbsp olive oil, organic

Preparation Steps: Sliced tomatoes have been washed. Combine basil, paprika, and cilantro. Stir well. Add the spice combination to the pressure cooker along with the tomato slices. Place a lid on after adding organic olive oil. The meal should be prepared slowly for 8 hours. The tomatoes must be semi-dry after the cooking process is finished. They must be taken out of the pressure cooker. Warm dried tomatoes should be served.

Nutritional Info: Calories: 92 kcal, Protein: 1g, Carb: 3.8g, Fat: 8.6g.

15.   Crunchy chicken skin

(Setup Time: 10 minutes | Cooked in: 10 minutes | How many people 7 | Difficulty: Easy)

Recipe Components:

- 1 tsp black pepper, ground
- 9 ozs of chicken skin
- 1 tsp of essential olive oil, organic
- 1 tsp of red chili flakes
- 1 tsp of salt
- 2 tbsp of butter
- 1 tsp of paprika

Preparation Steps: Combine paprika, chili flakes, and black pepper. Stir well all elements.

Chicken skin is added to the mixture and given five minutes to rest. Put butter in the pressure cooker's on sauté setting. The chicken skin should be added as soon as the butter melts, and it should be sautéed for 10 minutes with constant tossing. Take the chicken skin out of the pressure cooker when it becomes crispy and set it on the paper towel to absorb extra oil. Serve hot.

Nutritional Info: Calories: 134 kcal, Protein: 7g, Carb: 0.9g, Fat: 11.5g.

16. Ginger Cookies

(Setup Time: 10 minutes | Cooked in: 14 minutes | How many people 2 | Difficulty: Easy)

Recipe Components:

- 1 egg
- 3 tbsp. heavy cream
- 1 tsp. Ginger, ground
- ½ tsp. baking powder
- 1 cup almond flour
- 3 tbsp. Erythritol
- 3 tbsp. Butter
- ½ tsp. cinnamon, ground

Preparation Steps:

1. Gently whisk the egg into the bowl while beating it. Mix in the baking powder, ground cinnamon, erythritol, ginger, and heavy cream.

2. Mix the butter in carefully. We need to work on the dough, which is not sticky. Use a rolling pin to flatten out the cookie dough and a cookie cutter to cut out shapes for your cookies.

3. Put a single layer of cookies inside the basket and secure the cover. Bake the cookies for about 14 minutes at 350 degrees Fahrenheit.

4. Once the cookies are prepared, thoroughly cool them before serving!

Nutritional Info: Calories: 172 kcal, Protein: 4.4g, Carb: 4.1g, Fat: 15.6g.

17. Radish chips and pesto

(Setup Time: 10 minutes | Cooked in: 0 minutes | How many people 2 | Difficulty: Easy)

Recipe Components:

Pesto:

- 60 g or ⅓ heaping cup raw almonds, soaked in water for 12 hours, rinsed and drained
- 1 small clove of garlic
- 1 tbsp. apple cider vinegar
- ⅛ tsp sea salt, finely ground
- 60 g or 1 cup basil leaves, fresh

- 25 g or ⅓ cup fresh parsley stems and leaves
- 2 tbsp olive oil
- 1½ tsps lemon juice
- 3¼ oz./90 g 20 medium radishes, thinly sliced, to serve

Preparation Steps: Combine everything element to make the pesto in a powerful blender or food processor. Blend until smooth. To a serving dish, transfer the pesto. Serve the radishes once they have been cut into slices.

Nutritional Info: Calories: 337 kcal, Protein: 8.1g, Carb: 10.2g, Fat: 29.4g.

18. Dairy-Free Queso

(Setup Time: 10 minutes + 12 hours soaking | Cooked in: 10 minutes | How many people 5 | Difficulty: Hard)

Recipe Components:

- 120 ml or ½ cup nondairy milk
- ½ tsp sea salt, finely ground
- 1 yellow onion, medium sliced
- 1 tbsp. chili powder
- ¾ tsp garlic powder
- ½ tsp oregano leaves, dried
- ⅛ tsp cayenne pepper
- 130 g or 1 cup raw cashews
- 17 g or ¼ cup nutritional yeast
- 60 ml or ¼ cup avocado oil
- 2 cloves garlic, roughly chopped
- 1 tsp cumin, ground
- ¼ tsp onion powder
- ⅛ tsp paprika
- 100 g or 3½ ozs pork rinds and 2 medium zucchinis, chopped into sticks, to serve (optional)

Preparation Steps: Prepare a large, airtight jar to hold the cashews (at least 12 ozs/350 ml). Fill it with the water. To soak for 12 hours, cover and place the container in the fridge. After 12 hours, rinse the cashews under running water and add them to a food processor or blender along with the nutritional yeast, milk, and salt. Put away. In a large skillet, heat the oil until it shimmers over medium heat. After the garlic, onion, and spices have been added, toss in the onion. You should whisk the mixture every few minutes for about 10 minutes or until the onion softens. Put the onions and everything else in the blender or food processor. Mix it all together in a concealed blender. Pig rinds or zucchini sticks can be served with the queso.

Nutritional Info: Calories: 300 kcal, Protein: 6.5g, Carb: 11.3g, Fat: 24g.

Chapter 5: Vegan, Vegetable & Meatless Recipes

Below are the recipes.

1. Roasted Marinated mushrooms

(Setup Time: 10 minutes | Cooked in: 13 minutes | How many people: 6 | Difficulty: Easy)

Recipe Components:

- 1 onion
- 1-ounce bay leaf
- 3 tbsp apple cider vinegar
- 1 tsp of sea salt
- 10 ozs mushrooms
- 1 garlic clove
- ¼ tsp black-eyed peas
- 1 tbsp. olive oil
- 1 tsp black pepper, ground

Preparation Steps: Peel the garlic and onion cloves. Black-eyed peas are sliced and added to the veggies. Apple cider vinegar and bay leaf should be added. The mushrooms should be chopped and added to the onion mixture. Black pepper and sea salt should be added. Mix thoroughly, and then set aside for 10 minutes to rest. Set the sauté setting on the pressure cooker. Add all the mushroom mixture to the pressure cooker after adding the olive oil. Sauté the food for 13 minutes with your pressure cooker lid closed. Open your pressure cooker cover after the cooking period, and then mix well. Place the mushrooms in dishes for serving.

Nutritional Info: Calories: 189 kcal, Protein: 5g, Carb: 42.6g, Fat: 3.2g.

2. Ginger broccoli soup

(Setup Time: 5 minutes | Cooked in: 25 minutes | How many people: 4 | Difficulty: Easy)

Recipe Components:

- 1 white onion, small sliced
- 420 g or 5 cups broccoli florets
- 355 ml or 1½ cups chicken bone broth
- 1½ tsps turmeric powder
- 55 g or ⅓ cup collagen peptides (optional)
- 3 tbsp avocado or coconut oil
- 2 minced garlic cloves
- 400 ml 1 tin coconut milk, full-fat
- 2 inch 1 piece fresh ginger root, minced and peeled
- ¾ tsp sea salt, finely ground

- 40 g or ¼ cup sesame seeds

Preparation Steps: Melt the oil in a large frying pan over medium heat. Simmer the garlic and onion for about 10 minutes or until they are translucent. Broccoli, broth, coconut milk, ginger, salt, and turmeric should all be added. The broccoli should be soft after 15 minutes of cooking with the cover on. Add all broccoli mixture to a food processor or blender. If you're using collagen, mix it in thoroughly. Put in 4 bowls and top each with 1 tbsp. of the sesame seeds.

Nutritional Info: Calories: 344 kcal, Protein: 13.3g, Carb: 12.4g, Fat: 26.8g.

3. Sriracha carrots

(Setup Time: 10 minutes | Cooked in: 17 minutes | How many people: 7 | Difficulty: Easy)

Recipe Components:

- 1 cup of water
- 2 tbsp olive oil
- 1 pound carrots
- 2 tbsp sriracha
- 1 tsp Erythritol
- ½ cup dill
- 1 tsp oregano

Preparation Steps: The carrots should be washed, peeled, and sliced. Set the sauté setting on the pressure cooker. The pressure cooker should be filled with olive oil before adding the carrot slices. Add some dill and oregano to the veggies. Stirring often throughout the 15 minutes of sautéing the food. Add water, erythritol, and sriracha to the carrot. Mix thoroughly. Cook the food on Pressure mode for about 2 minutes with the pressure cooker lid closed. Release any leftover pressure to open the pressure cooker lid when the cooking step is complete. Onto a serving platter, place the carrots.

Nutritional Info: Calories: 74 kcal, Protein: 1.2g, Carb: 9.3g, Fat: 4.2g.

4. Roasted veggie mix

(Setup Time: 10 minutes | Cooked in: 30 minutes | How many people: 10 | Difficulty: Easy)

Recipe Components:

- 2 yellow bell peppers
- 8 ozs tomatoes
- 1 zucchini
- 2 carrots
- 4 cups beef broth
- 2 eggplants
- 1 tbsp. salt
- 2 turnips
- 1 tbsp. oregano
- 3 tbsp sesame oil

Preparation Steps: Chop the eggplants after peeling them. Salt the eggplants, then thoroughly stir. Bell peppers with seeds removed should be chopped. Chop the turnips and slice the tomatoes. Slice the zucchini. Grate the carrots after peeling them. All the veggies should be added to your pressure cooker. Add the beef broth, sesame oil, and oregano.

Stir well, and then secure the pressure cooker cover. For thirty minutes, steam the meal. Transfer the meal to serving dishes after the cooking period is over.

Nutritional Info: Calories: 107 kcal, Protein: 4g, Carb: 13.2g, Fat: 5g.

5. Cauliflower puree with scallions

(Setup Time: 15 minutes | Cooked in: 7 minutes | How many people: 6 | Difficulty: Easy)

Recipe Components:

4 cups of water

- 4 tbsp butter
- 1 tsp chicken stock
- 1 egg yolk

- 1 head cauliflower
- 1 tbsp. salt
- 3 ozs scallions
- ¼ tsp sesame seeds

Preparation Steps: Cauliflower should be washed and roughly chopped. In the pressure cooker, put the cauliflower. Salt and water are added. Vegetables should be cooked in pressure mode for about 5 minutes with the lid closed. Open your pressure cooker cover to let the pressure out. Cauliflower should be removed from the pressure cooker and given time to rest. Blend the cauliflower in a food processor. Chicken stock, butter, and sesame seeds should be added. The substance has been well blended. Slice the scallions. Blend the mixture in the blender for 30 seconds after adding the egg yolk. The scallions should be added to the cauliflower puree after removing it from the blender. Mix thoroughly, then plate.

Nutritional Info: Calories: 94 kcal, Protein: 2g, Carb: 3.4g, Fat: 8.7g.

6. Spinach Quiche

(Setup Time: 10 minutes | Cooked in: 33 minutes | How many people: 4 | Difficulty: Easy)

Recipe Components:

- 1 pack of spinach, frozen and thawed
- Salt and pepper to taste
- 1 tbsp. melted butter

- 5 beaten eggs, organic
- 3 cups shredded Monterey Jack Cheese

Preparation Steps: Set the Ninja Foodi to Sauté mode and wait for it to warm up before adding butter and allowing it to melt. Spinach should be added and cooked for three minutes before being removed and placed in a serving bowl. Beat eggs and add to bowl with cheese, seasonings, and pepper. Put the mixture into greased quiche shapes and pop them into your Foodi. Close the cover, choose "Bake/Roast," and cook for about 30 minutes at 360 degrees Fahrenheit. Open the cover when finished, and then remove the dish. Serve after cutting into wedges.

Nutritional Info: Calories: 349 kcal, Protein: 23g, Carb: 3.2g, Fat: 27g.

7. Brussels sprouts

(Setup Time: 7 minutes | Cooked in: 4 minutes | How many people: 6 | Difficulty: Easy)

Recipe Components:

- 1 tsp salt
- ½ tsp coriander
- 1 cup chicken stock
- 1 tbsp. butter
- 13 ozs Brussels sprouts
- 1 tsp cumin
- ½ tsp chili powder
- 1 tsp thyme
- 1 tsp olive oil

Preparation Steps: After cleaning, add the Brussels sprouts to the pressure cooker. Salt, coriander, cumin, thyme, and chili powder combine and well mixed. After thoroughly stirring, sprinkle the spice mixture over the Brussels sprouts. Add chicken stock, butter, and olive oil. Select Pressure mode on the pressure cooker. Snap the pressure cooker's lid shut. For 4 minutes, cook at. Release all pressure and open your pressure cooker cover when cooking is complete. Put the prepared food in dishes for serving.

Nutritional Info: Calories: 67 kcal, Protein: 3g, Carb: 7.2g, Fat: 3.5g.

8. Kale salad with spicy lime-tahini dressing

(Setup Time: 15 minutes | Cooked in: 0 minutes | How many people: 4 | Difficulty: Easy)

Recipe Components:

Salad:

- 12 radishes, thinly sliced
- 1 medium Hass avocado, pitted, peeled, and cubed
- 360 g or 6 cups de-stemmed kale leaves, roughly chopped
- 1 sliced green bell pepper
- 30 g or ¼ cup hulled pumpkin seeds

Dressing:

- 60 ml or ¼ cup lime juice
- 2 minced cloves garlic
- Handful of freshly chopped cilantro leaves
- ½ tsp sea salt, finely ground
- 120 ml or ½ cup avocado oil
- 60 ml or ¼ cup tahini
- 1 jalapeño pepper, finely diced and seeded

- ½ tsp cumin, ground
- ¼ tsp red pepper flakes

Preparation Steps: Mix all ingredients inside a medium bowl using a whisk to prepare the dressing. Place aside. Assemble the salad: To soften and make the kale simpler to digest, rinse it in hot water for approximately 30 seconds. Place the kale in a big salad dish after thoroughly drying it. Toss in the leftover salad ingredients after adding them. Four bowls should get an equal amount of salad. Pour 14 cups (60 ml) of your dressing into each bowl before serving.

RETAIN IT: For up to five days, store the salad and dressing in different airtight containers inside the refrigerator. The avocado should not be added to your recipe until just before serving.

Nutritional Info: Calories: 517 kcal, Protein: 10.7g, Carb: 21g, Fat: 47g.

9. Vegetable tart

(Setup Time: 15 minutes | Cooked in: 25 minutes | How many people: 9 | Difficulty: Moderate)

Recipe Components:

- 1 egg yolk
- 5 ozs tomatoes
- 1 eggplant
- 1 tsp salt
- 1 tsp black pepper, ground
- 7 ozs of goat cheese
- 7 ozs puff pastry
- 2 red bell peppers
- 1 red onion
- 3 ozs zucchini
- 1 tsp olive oil
- 1 tbsp. turmeric
- ¼ cup cream

Preparation Steps: Black pepper and egg yolk are thoroughly combined after whisking. A rolling pin is used to roll the puff pastry. Spray some olive oil into the pressure cooker, and then add all-puff pastry. The whisked egg should be spread over the puff pastry. Cut the onions and tomatoes into dice. Slice the zucchini and eggplant. After combining the veggies, season them with turmeric, salt, and cream. After thoroughly combining, add the vegetable mixture to the pressure cooker. Red bell peppers should be chopped and added to the pressure cooker mixture. Grate the goat cheese, and then top the tart with it. Snap the pressure cooker's lid shut. Cook for 25 minutes in pressure mode. Release all pressure and open your pressure cooker cover after the food is done. Once the tart has been thoroughly cooked, take it from your pressure cooker. Serve the tart by cutting it into wedges.

Nutritional Info: Calories: 279 kcal, Protein: 10g, Carb: 18.4g, Fat: 18.8g.

10. Stewed cabbage

(Setup Time: 10 minutes | Cooked in: 30 minutes | How many people: 7 | Difficulty: Easy)

Recipe Components:

- 2 red bell pepper
- 1 cup tomato juice
- 1 tsp salt
- 1 tsp basil
- 13 ozs cabbage
- ¼ chile pepper
- 1 tbsp. olive oil
- 1 tsp paprika
- ½ cup chopped dill

Preparation Steps: The cabbage should be washed and cut into small pieces. Use your hands to thoroughly combine the paprika, salt, and basil with the chopped cabbage. Place the pressure cooker with the chopped cabbage inside. Olive oil, tomato juice, and chopped dill should all be added Red bell pepper and chile pepper should be chopped. Mix thoroughly before adding the veggies to the pressure cooker. Cook the meal on "Sauté" mode for 30 minutes with your pressure cooker lid closed. Once the food has finished cooking, serve it after a little rest.

Nutritional Info: Calories: 46 kcal, Protein: 1g, Carb: 6.6g, Fat: 2.2g.

11. Zucchini pizza

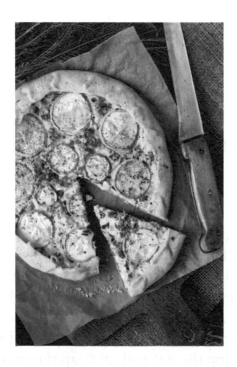

(Setup Time: 10 minutes | Cooked in: 8 minutes | How many people: 2 | Difficulty: Easy)

Recipe Components:

- ½ tsp tomato paste
- ½ tsp chili flakes
- 1 tsp olive oil
- 1 zucchini
- 5 oz. Parmesan, shredded
- ¼ tsp basil, dried

Preparation Steps: For boards, cut your zucchini in half. Then, remove the meat from the inside and smear it with tomato paste. After that, stuff zucchini with cheese shreds. Olive oil, dried basil, and chili flakes are sprinkled on them.

Pizzas made with zucchini should be placed inside the oven with the cover on. Pizzas should be baked for 8 minutes at 375 degrees F in crisp air mode.

Nutritional Info: Calories: 331 kcal, Protein: 28.1g, Carb: 6g, Fat: 21.9g.

12. Spicy Cauliflower Steak

(Setup Time: 10 minutes | Cooked in: 4 minutes | How many people: 6 | Difficulty: Easy)

Recipe Components:

- 2 tbsp olive oil, extra-virgin
- 2 tsp ground cumin
- 1 cup fresh chopped cilantro
- 1 large head of cauliflower
- 2 tsps paprika
- ¾ tsp kosher salt
- 1 lemon, quartered

Preparation Steps: The steamer rack should be put into the Ninja Foodi. Include 1.5 cups of water. Cauliflower's leaves should be removed, and the center should be trimmed to sit flat. Carefully position it on the steam rack. Get a small bowl and fill it with salt, cumin, paprika, and olive oil. Pour the sauce over the cauliflower. Put the lid back on and let the pressure cook for 4 minutes. Release the pressure quickly. Slice the cauliflower into 1-inch steaks after transferring it to a cutting board. Place a portion of the mixture on each dish, then top with cilantro. Dispense and savor!

Nutritional Info: Calories: 283 kcal, Protein: 10g, Carb: 18g, Fat: 19g.

Chapter 6: Pork, Beef, Lamb & Poultry Recipes

Below are the recipes.

1. Chicken and Cabbage Meatball

(Setup Time: 7 minutes | Cooked in: 4 minutes | How many people: 4 | Difficulty: Easy)

Recipe Components:

- ¼ cup heavy whipped cream
- ½ tsp caraway seeds, ground
- ¼ tsp allspice, ground
- ½ cup almond milk
- 1 lb. chicken, ground
- 2 tsps salt
- 1½ tsps black pepper, ground and divided
- 4 to 6 cups chopped green cabbage
- 2 tbsp butter, unsalted

Preparation Steps: Place the meat in a bowl. Cream, 1 tsp salt, 1/2 tsp pepper, caraway, and allspice should be mixed together completely. Put the mixture in the fridge for 30 minutes. Scoop all mixture into the meatballs after cooling. Add half the balls and half the cabbage to the Ninja Foodi pot. Add the remaining balls, and then top with the rest of the cabbage. Add milk, butter pats, and a sprinkling. 1 tsp each of salt and pepper. Put the cover on and cook under high pressure for 4 minutes. A rapid release of pressure. Lock the lid, and then serve.

Nutritional Info: Calories: 294 kcal, Protein: 12g, Carb: 4g, Fat: 26g.

2. BBQ Chicken

(Setup Time: 5 minutes | Cooked in: 17 minutes | How many people: 6 | Difficulty: Easy)

Recipe Components:

- 1 tbsp. olive oil
- ¼ tsp. black pepper
- 1 cup hot sauce
- 2 tbsp vinegar
- 1½ lbs. chicken thighs, skinless and boneless
- 1 tsp. paprika, ground
- 1 onion, chopped
- ¼ cup water

Preparation Steps: Put some olive oil in the Ninja Foodi and turn it into the sauté mode. The chicken thighs should be cooked for 2 minutes per side after being added. Season the chicken with salt and pepper, then throw everything else into the pot with it. Cover the Ninja Foodi and cook the chicken for 15 minutes on high heat using the pressure cooker mode. Use the steam release method to release pressure, and then use two forks to shred the chicken. You may serve it hot or cold.

Nutritional Info: Calories: 215 kcal, Protein: 17g, Carb: 1g, Fat: 16g

3. Crispy thighs and mash

(Setup Time: 15 minutes | Cooked in: 30 minutes | How many people: 6 | Difficulty: Easy)

Recipe Components:

Crispy Chicken:

- 60 ml or ¼ cup coconut oil or avocado oil, melted
- ½ tsp onion powder
- ¼ tsp black pepper, ground
- 1 lb. 3 large or 6 small skinless and boneless chicken thighs
- 1 tsp garlic powder
- ¼ tsp sea salt, finely ground

Butternut Mash:

- 2 tbsp coconut ghee or oil
- ⅛ Tsp black pepper, ground
- 1½ tbsp chicken bone broth
- 1¼ lbs. 1 medium butternut squash
- ½ tsp sea salt, finely ground
- 80 ml or ⅓ cup milk (regular or non-dairy)

Preparation Steps: Prepare the chicken: Set the oven's temperature to 400°F (205°C). Cut big chicken thighs in half to create 6 pieces if using them. On a baking sheet with a rim, arrange the chicken. The thighs are covered in oil, then the spices are sprinkled on top. The thighs should be turned to evenly distribute the oil and seasoning. To ensure an internal temperature of 165 degrees Fahrenheit (74 degrees Celsius), bake the chicken for 25 to 30 minutes. Slice the chicken into 1.25 cm-thick (1.12 inch) pieces. Make the mash in the interim: Cut the squash's meat into cubes after removing the peel and seeds. Measure out 3 cups (455 g) of your squash cubes for the mash; save the rest for another use by storing it in the refrigerator. The oil is heated in a large frying pan over medium heat. Mix in the seasonings and the squash. After 10-15 minutes of covered cooking, the squash should be lightly caramelized. Once the squash has reached a softness that allows for mashing, add the milk and broth, cover, and continue boiling for 15 minutes. Using the back of a fork, mash the squash in the pan once it's done cooking. Divide the mash over 6 dinner plates to serve. Enjoy! Place an equal quantity of all sliced chicken thighs on each serving.

Nutritional Info: Calories: 331 kcal, Protein: 16.2g, Carb: 9.9g, Fat: 26.5g.

4. Keto-Friendly Chicken Tortillas

(Setup Time: 7 minutes | Cooked in: 15 minutes | How many people: 4 | Difficulty: Easy)

Recipe Components:

- 1 lb. boneless chicken breasts, pastured organic
- 2 tsps. Worcestershire sauce, gluten-free

- 1 tsp. Salt
- ½ tsp. paprika
- 1 tbsp. avocado oil
- ½ cup orange juice
- 1 tsp. garlic powder
- ½ tsp. chili powder

Preparation Steps: Put your Ninja Foodi in sauté mode, add some oil, and then wait for it to warm up. Put the chicken in a bowl and mix in the rest of the ingredients. Pour the sauce over the chicken. Cook for 15 minutes at high pressure with the lid on. Over ten minutes, naturally release the pressure. Chicken should be shredded with green salad, lettuce or cabbage.

Nutritional Info: Calories: 338 kcal, Protein: 23g, Carb: 10g, Fat: 23g.

5. Hot Spicy Paprika Chicken

(Setup Time: 10 minutes | Cooked in: 24 minutes | How many people: 4 | Difficulty: Easy)

Recipe Components:

- Pepper and salt
- ½ cup sweet onion, chopped
- 2 tsps paprika, smoked
- 2 tbsp parsley, chopped
- 4 pieces of chicken breast
- 1 tbsp. olive oil
- ½ cup heavy whipped cream
- ½ cup sour cream

Preparation Steps: Lightly season the chicken with pepper and salt. Put your Ninja Foodi in sauté mode, add some oil, and then wait for it to warm up. It will take around 15 minutes to sear the chicken on both sides after you add it. Chicken should be taken out and placed on a platter. Saute an onion in a pan for 4 minutes, or until tender, over medium heat; then, add cream and paprika and bring to a boil. Add the chicken back to the skillet, along with any juices. Place the cover on the Ninja Foodi and cook the whole mixture for 5 minutes at high pressure. Over ten minutes, naturally release the pressure. Sour cream has been added; serve and enjoy!

Nutritional Info: Calories: 389 kcal, Protein: 25g, Carb: 4g, Fat: 30g.

6. Cream of Mushroom–Stuffed Chicken

(Setup Time: 10 minutes | Cooked in: 45 minutes | How many people: 4 | Difficulty: Easy)

Recipe Components:

- 200 g or 7 ozs cremini mushrooms, chopped
- 3 tsps parsley, dried and divided
- ¼ tsp black pepper, ground
- 1 tsp onion powder
- 120 ml or ½ cup milk (regular or non-dairy)
- 3 tbsp avocado oil, coconut oil, or ghee
- 4 cloves garlic, minced

- ¾ tsp sea salt, divided and finely ground

- 455 g or 1 pound skin-on chicken breasts, boneless

- 1 tsp garlic powder

- 280 g or 4 cups spinach to serve

Preparation Steps: Warm up the oven to 400 degrees Fahrenheit (205 degrees C). Use a silicone baking mat or parchment paper to line a rimmed baking sheet. Heat the oil in a large frying pan over medium heat. Combine the mushrooms with 2 tsps of parsley, 1 clove of garlic, 1/4 tsp of salt, and a few grinds of black pepper. Sauté for 10 minutes after coating and stirring. To open each chicken breast like a book, slice it horizontally, halting the knife about ½ inch (1.25 cm) via the other side. Be cautious not to cut through the chicken breasts completely. The easiest technique is with a sharp knife, holding it stable with your hand on the breast. Open the chicken breasts and place them on the prepared baking sheet. Each opened breast should have a quarter of your mushroom mixture inside the center. Scatter any remaining mushroom mixture in the pan next to the chicken. To enclose the filling, fold the chicken breasts over. Garlic powder, the last tsp of parsley, onion powder, and the last tsp of salt should all be sprinkled over the filled chicken breasts. Directly into the pan, pour the milk in the space between the chicken breasts. Make sure the chicken achieves an internal temperature of 165 degrees Fahrenheit (74 degrees Celsius) by baking it for 30 to 35 minutes. 4 dinner plates should each get some spinach. On each dish, distribute the filled chicken breasts. Drizzle all spinach using the rich pan juices. Note: Divide the stuffed breasts into parts and serve them on equal numbers of plates. If you don't wind up with 1 breast, half every person in the packet.

Nutritional Info: Calories: 388 kcal, Protein: 38.2g, Carb: 4.3g, Fat: 24.3g.

7. Chili Rubbed Chicken

(Setup Time: 10 minutes | Cooked in: 30 minutes | How many people: 2 | Difficulty: Easy)

Recipe Components:

- 1 tbsp. chili powder
- Ground black pepper, to taste
- 1 tsp. garlic powder
- 2 chicken thighs
- 1 tbsp. Paprika

- 2 tbsp salt
- 1 tsp. Onion powder
- 1 tsp. cumin, ground
- 1 tbsp. olive oil

Preparation Steps: Combine all the spices in a bowl and then put it aside. Olive oil should be used to coat the chicken thighs before being seasoned. Turn your Ninja Foodi to 375 degrees, add the spiced chicken to the cook and crisp basket, and finish cooking. Set the timer for about 30 minutes and place the basket into the Ninja Foodi. Serve when still heated.

Nutritional Info: Calories: 230 kcal, Protein: 15g, Carb: 7g, Fat: 16g.

8. BBQ beef and slaw

(Setup Time: 10 minutes | Cooked in: 45 minutes (4 to 6 hours additional) | How many people: 4 | Difficulty: Moderate)

Recipe Components:

BBQ Beef:

- 240 ml or 1 cup beef bone broth
- 80 g or ½ cup barbecue sauce, sugar-free
- 455 g or 1 pound beef chuck roast, boneless
- ½ tsp sea salt, finely ground

Slaw:

- 120 ml or ½ cup poppy seed dressing, sugar-free
- 255 g or 9 ozs coleslaw mix

Preparation Steps: A slow or pressure cooker should include the chuck roast, stock, and salt. Secure the cover and cook for 45 minutes at high pressure if utilizing a pressure cooker. Let the lid come off naturally when everything is finished to escape the pressure. For a slow cooker, set the timer for 4 hours on high or 6 hours on low. After the meat is cooked, almost all the liquid should be drained away, leaving just about 1/4 cup (60 ml) in the cooker. Shred the pork using two forks, then add the barbecue sauce and stir to blend. In a salad dish, combine all coleslaw mix and dressing. Toss to combine. Enjoy the barbecued beef and coleslaw by dividing them among four dinner plates, putting the steak on the bottom and the coleslaw on top.

Nutritional Info: Calories: 354 kcal, Protein: 23.9g, Carb: 2.9g, Fat: 26.7g.

9. Coffee Braised Pulled Beef

(Setup Time: 15 minutes | Cooked in: 35 minutes | How many people: 6 | Difficulty: Hard)

Recipe Components:

For Rub:

- 1 tbsp. cacao powder
- 1 tsp ginger, ground
- 1 tsp crushed red pepper flakes
- 2 pounds beef chuck roast grass-fed, trimmed and chopped into 1½-inch cubes
- 2 tbsp finely ground coffee
- 1 tbsp. paprika, smoked
- 1 tsp red chili powder
- Salt and ground black pepper

For Sauce:

- ½ cup brewed coffee
- 2 tbsp lemon juice, fresh
- 1 cup beef broth, homemade
- 1 yellow onion, medium chopped
- Salt and ground black pepper, as needed

Preparation Steps: Except for the roast, mix all the rub ingredients together in a small basin. Use a lot of the rub mixture to coat the chuck roast. Put all the sauce components into a food processor and blitz until smooth; that's how you make sauce. Place the roast in the Ninja Foodi pot and evenly distribute the sauce on top. Put the pressure lid on the Ninja Foodi and turn the pressure valve to the Seal position to close it. Select High Pressure and cook for 35 minutes. To start cooking, click Start/Stop. Put the valve on the Vent, then release naturally. Put the roast in a basin and shred the flesh with two forks. Add the pot sauce on top before serving.

Nutritional Info: Calories: 573 kcal, Protein: 41.1g, Carb: 3.7g, Fat: 42.8g.

10. Beef Jerky

(Setup Time: 15 minutes | Cooked in: 7 hours | How many people: 6 | Difficulty: Moderate)

Recipe Components:

- 2 tbsp. Worcestershire sauce
- Salt, as needed
- ¼ cup soy sauce, low-sodium
- 2 tbsp. Erythritol
- 1½ pounds beef eye of round grass-fed, cut in ¼-inch slices

Preparation Steps: Put all the ingredients in a bowl—aside from the beef— and beat until the sugar completely dissolves. Place the beef pieces and marinate in a large plastic bag that can be sealed. To coat, seal your bag and massage. Overnight marinating in the refrigerator. After removing the beef slices from the refrigerator, drain them and throw away the marinade. Put the beef slices in a single layer in the Cook & Crisp Basket. In the Ninja Foodi pot, arrange the Cook & Crisp Basket. Select Dehydrate and close your Ninja Foodi with Crisping Lid. Set the thermostat to 155 degrees Fahrenheit for seven hours. To start cooking, click Start/Stop.

Nutritional Info: Calories: 199 kcal, Protein: 33.5g, Carb: 1.7g, Fat: 5.6g.

11. Spicy Pulled Beef

(Setup Time: 15 minutes | Cooked in: 1 hour 30 minutes | How many people: 10 | Difficulty: Hard)

Recipe Components:

- 5 peeled garlic cloves
- 2 tbsp lime juice, fresh
- 1 tbsp. cumin, ground
- ½ tsp cloves, ground

- 3 pounds beef bottom round roast grass-fed, trimmed and chopped into 3-inch pieces
- 1 tsp olive oil
- ½ onion, medium
- 3 tbsp chipotles inside adobo sauce
- 1 tbsp. oregano, dried and crushed
- ½ tsp cayenne pepper
- 1 cup water
- Salt and ground black pepper
- 3 bay leaves

Preparation Steps: Until smooth, combine onion, chipotles, garlic, lime juice, cumin, oregano, cayenne, and cloves in a blender with the water. Evenly sprinkle black pepper and salt over the meat. Place all oil in the pot and choose Ninja Foodi's Sauté/Sear option. To start cooking and heat for around 2-3 minutes, press Start/Stop. When the meat is thoroughly browned, add it and simmer for approximately 5 minutes. After stopping the cooking by pressing Start/Stop, toss in your pureed mixture and bay leaves. Put the pressure lid on the Ninja Foodi and turn the pressure valve to the Seal position to close it. Select High Pressure and cook for 65 minutes. To start cooking, click Start/Stop. Change the valve's setting to Vent and perform a quick release. Using a slotted spoon, put the meat in a bowl, and then use two forks to shred it. Stir and add 1 ½ cups of the liquid that was set aside. Serve right away.

Nutritional Info: Calories: 266 kcal, Protein: 41.6g, Carb: 1.8g, Fat: 9.2g.

12. Bacon Wrapped Beef Tenderloins

(Setup Time: 15 minutes | Cooked in: 12 minutes | How many people: 4 | Difficulty: Moderate)

Recipe Components:

- 4 grass-fed beef tenderloin filets, center-cut
- Salt and ground black pepper
- 8 bacon strips
- 2 tbsp divided olive oil

Preparation Steps: Secure each filet with toothpicks. Each filet should be uniformly seasoned with black pepper and salt after being oil-coated. Put the Reversible Rack into the Ninja Foodi pot. Select Broil for 5 minutes while the Ninja Foodi with Crisping Lid is closed. For the preheating to start, press Start/Stop. Open the cover after preheating. Over the Reversible Rack, arrange the beef filets. With the crisping lid closed, choose Broil for about 12 minutes. To start cooking, click Start/Stop. Once they are halfway done, flip the filets. Before serving, spread the filets on a plate for approximately 10 minutes. Each beef filet should have 2 bacon strips wrapped around the outside of it.

Nutritional Info: Calories: 841 kcal, Protein: 87g, Carb: 0.8g, Fat: 52g.6)

13. Fajita Beef

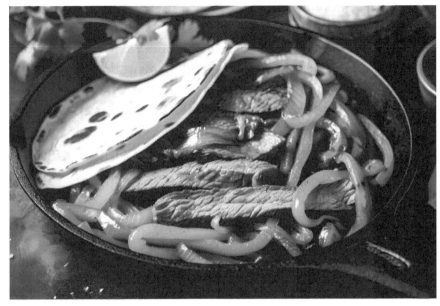

(Setup Time: 7 minutes | Cooked in: 7 hours | How many people: 4 | Difficulty: Easy)

Recipe Components:

- 3 bell peppers, sliced and seeded
- 2 pounds of boneless grass-fed beef, sliced
- ½ tin diced tomatoes with green chiles, sugar-free
- 2 tbsp butter
- 1 yellow sliced onion
- 2 tbsp fajita seasoning

Preparation Steps: Place your butter in the saucepan and choose the Sauté/Sear mode on Ninja Foodi. To start cooking and heat for around 2-3 minutes, press Start/Stop.

Cook the onion and bell pepper for two to three minutes after adding them. After adding the fajita spice, cook the meat for 4-5 minutes. To stop cooking and then stir in the tomato can, press Start/Stop. Select Slow Cooker, and then close your Ninja Foodi with a crisping cover. Set for seven hours on low. To start cooking, click Start/Stop. Serve warm.

Nutritional Info: Calories: 658 kcal, Protein: 22.5g, Carb: 6.1g, Fat: 58.9g.

14. The Premium Red Pork

(Setup Time: 10 minutes | Cooked in: 40 minutes | How many people: 6 | Difficulty: Moderate)

Recipe Components:

- 2 tbsp maple syrup
- 1 tbsp. blackstrap molasses
- 1 tsp salt
- 1-piece ginger, smashed and peeled
- 2 pounds of pork belly
- 3 tbsp sherry
- 2 tbsp coconut amino
- 1/3 cup water

- A few sprigs of cilantro for garnishing

Preparation Steps: Over medium heat, place the pork in a saucepan with enough water to cover. Give the water a chance to boil. Drain and clean the ice cubes after three minutes of boiling to eliminate contaminants. Place them on one side. Sauté mode on your Ninja Foodi, then add maple syrup. Add the cooked cubes and brown them for one minute. Add the ingredients to the stew after 10 minutes, and then bring the whole mixture to a boil. Cook for about 25 minutes at high pressure with the lid closed. Allow all pressure to decrease naturally. Open the lid and go back to Sauté mode on your Ninja Foodi. Simmer the mixture once enough liquid is reduced to coat the ice cubes. Serve with cilantro as a garnish. Enjoy!

Nutritional Info: Calories: 355 kcal, Protein: 31g, Carb: 16g, Fat: 13g.

15. Crispy Pork with thyme-lemon cauliflower rice

(Setup Time: 5 minutes | Cooked in: 40 minutes | How many people: 4 | Difficulty: Moderate)

Recipe Components:

Crispy Pork:

- 38 g or ½ cup pork rinds, crushed
- 1 tsp oregano leaves, dried
- ½ tsp sea salt, finely ground
- 455 g or 1 pound pork chops, boneless
- 55 g or ¼ cup coconut ghee or oil, or 60 ml ¼ cup avocado oil
- 1 tsp garlic powder
- 1 tsp thyme leaves, dried
- ¼ tsp black pepper, ground

Thyme-Lemon Cauliflower Rice:

- 1 white onion, small diced
- 60 ml or ¼ cup chicken bone broth
- ½ tsp sea salt, finely ground
- 680 g or 1½ lbs. 1 medium head cauliflower, or 3 cups (375 g) cauliflower, pre-riced
- 4 minced cloves of garlic
- 2 tbsp lemon juice
- 6 sprigs leaves of fresh thyme

Preparation Steps: Prepare the oil by heating it in a large frying pan over low to medium heat. In a medium bowl, mix the crushed pork rinds with the oregano, garlic powder, salt, thyme, and pepper while the oil is heating. One at a time, add all pork chops and coat them in the mixture after stirring to combine. Transfer the chops to your frying pan after they are well coated.

The pork chops should be properly seared after 10 minutes on each side. Use pre-riced cauliflower and go on to Step 5 instead. Otherwise, trim the cauliflower's base off and separate the florets. The florets should be placed in a blender or food processor and pulsed three to four times to create pieces that are 1/4 inch (6 mm) in size. Transfer all chops to a clean dish when the pork has cooked for 20 minutes, but keep the cooking oil in the pan. Add the broth, salted lemon juiced and riced cauliflower. Approximately 15 minutes of cooking should be allotted for the cauliflower rice to become soft yet not mushy while stirring occasionally. Slice all pork chops into 12-inch (1.25-cm) thick pieces as you wait. Add the sliced pork into the skillet after the cauliflower rice is cooked. Cook the pork uncovered for 5 minutes if necessary to ensure complete cooking. On 4 dinner plates, distribute the cauliflower rice and pork. Garnish with thyme leaves.

Nutritional Info: Calories: 419 kcal, Protein: 34g, Carb: 6g, Fat: 27.7g.

16. Butter and Dill Pork Chops

(Setup Time: 10 minutes | Cooked in: 20 minutes | How many people: 4 | Difficulty: Easy)

Recipe Components:

- 4 pieces pork loin chops, ½ inch thick
- ½ tsp pepper
- ½ cup white wine vinegar
- 2 tbsp butter, unsalted
- ½ tsp salt
- 16 baby carrots
- ½ cup chicken broth

Preparation Steps: Set the Sauté mode on your Ninja Foodi. Sprinkle salt and pepper on the chops. Chops should be thrown into a saucepan and cooked for four minutes. Cook and brown the remaining chops before transferring the first batch to a dish. 1 tbsp. of butter should be added. Put the dill and carrots in the cooker and heat for approximately a minute. When the stock begins to boil, add all of the wine and remove any browned bits from the pot's bottom. Add the broth and stir. Bring the chops back to your pot. Lock the cover and cook it under high pressure for about 18 minutes. Of course, let the pressure out by leaving it alone for 8 minutes. Open, and then serve using some sauce on top.

Nutritional Info: Calories: 296 kcal, Protein: 17g, Carb: 2g, Fat: 25g.

17. Happy Burrito Bowl Pork

(Setup Time: 10 minutes | Cooked in: 5 minutes | How many people: 4 | Difficulty: Easy)

Recipe Components:

- 1 sliced onion
- 1 chopped garlic clove
- 1 pound pulled pork
- ½ cup chicken broth
- 6 cups chopped cabbage
- 1 and ½ tbsp pork lard
- 2 sliced bell peppers
- Salt and pepper to taste

- ½ cup of chicken pork
- 6 cups chopped lettuce
- ¼ cup guacamole

Preparation Steps: Melt the lard in the Ninja Foodi on the Sauté mode, then add the onion and bell pepper. Stir constantly for two minutes as the food cooks. Salt, Garlic, and pepper are added. Stir well. Add chicken pork and pulled pork. Lock the cover and cook for one minute under high pressure. A rapid release of pressure. Put green cabbage and lettuce in serving dishes, and then top with pulled pork. Serve after adding guacamole on top. Enjoy!

Nutritional Info: Calories: 417 kcal, Protein: 75g, Carb: 6g, Fat: 95g.

18. Pork Carnitas

(Setup Time: 10 minutes | Cooked in: 25 minutes | How many people: 4 | Difficulty: Easy)

Recipe Components:

- 1 tsp salt
- ½ tsp cumin
- 6 garlic cloves, crushed and peeled
- 2 pounds pork butt, chopped into 2-inch pieces
- ½ tsp oregano
- 1 yellow onion, cut into half
- ½ cup chicken broth

Preparation Steps: Put the pork in a pan in your Ninja Foodi. Make sure the pork is well-seasoned by adding cumin, salt, and oregano and mixing thoroughly. Add the squeezed orange to the insert pan after taking the orange and squeezing it all over it. Add the onions and garlic cloves. Fill the pan with 1/2 cup of chicken broth. Lock the Ninja Foodi's lid, ensuring the valve is well secured. Set the pressure to high and let it 20 minutes to cook. Release the pressure immediately once the timer sounds. Remove the orange, the onions, and the garlic cloves by opening the lid. Set the temperature on the Nina Foodi to medium-high and choose the Sauté option. Simmer the liquid for ten to fifteen minutes. Press the stop button once most of your liquid has been decreased. Close the "Air Crisp" cover on the Ninja Foodi. Choose "Pressure Broil" and set the timer for 8 minutes. Put the meat in wrappers after taking it out. Enjoy with cilantro as a garnish!

Nutritional Info: Calories: 355 kcal, Protein: 43g, Carb: 9g, Fat: 13g.

19. Ham-Stuffed Turkey Rolls

(Setup Time: 8 minutes | Cooked in: 20 minutes | How many people: 8 | Difficulty: Easy)

Recipe Components:

- 8 ham slices
- Salt and pepper
- 4 tbsp sage leaves, fresh
- 8 turkey cutlets
- 2 tbsp butter, melted

Preparation Steps: Salt and pepper turkey cutlets before serving. Each turkey cutlet is securely wrapped in ham slices after being rolled. Butter each roll and delicately arrange sage leaves on top of each cutlet. You may bake them in a Ninja Foodi for 10 minutes at 360 degrees Fahrenheit by placing on the lid, selecting "Bake/Roast," and turning on the appliance. Lock the cover again and bake for 10 minutes after gently flipping it. Serve and savor once finished!

Nutritional Info: Calories: 467 kcal, Protein: 56g, Carb: 1.7g, Fat: 24g.

20. Turkey Cutlets

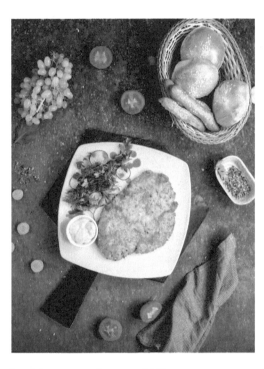

(Setup Time: 10 minutes | Cooked in: 22 minutes | How many people: 4 | Difficulty: Easy)

Recipe Components:

- 1 lb. turkey cutlets
- 1 tsp. turmeric powder
- 1 tsp. Greek seasoning
- 2 tsps olive oil
- ½ cup almond flour

Preparation Steps: Greek seasoning, almond flour, and turmeric powder should all be combined in a bowl. Turkey cutlets should be dredged in the basin and let soak for 30 minutes. Set your Ninja Foodi to Sauté mode, add oil, and let it warm up. Add cutlets, and then cook for two minutes. Lock the cover and cook for 20 minutes at low-medium pressure. Over ten minutes, naturally release the pressure. Remove the dish, serve, and enjoy!

Nutritional Info: Calories: 340 kcal, Protein: 36g, Carb: 3.7g, Fat: 19g.

Chapter 7: Fish & Seafood Recipes

Below are the recipes.

1. Salmon and Kale

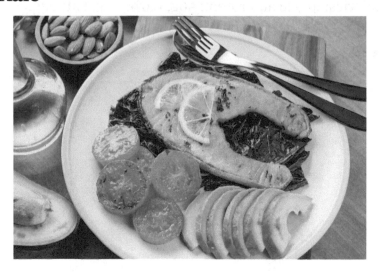

(Setup Time: 5 minutes + 2 hours marinating | Cooked in: 15 minutes | How many people: 4 | Difficulty: Easy)

Recipe Components:

- 180 ml or ¾ cup vinaigrette of choice
- 240 g or 4 cups de-stemmed kale leaves
- ¼ tsp sea salt, finely ground

- 455 g or 1 pound salmon fillets chopped into 4 equal portions
- 1 red onion, small sliced
- ¼ tsp red pepper flakes

Preparation Steps: In a small bowl, toss the salmon with the vinaigrette. For two hours of marinating, place covered in the refrigerator. When cooking, toss the salmon and all of the marinade ingredients into a large frying pan. Make a circle with the fish and turn the heat down to medium or low. Salmon should be cooked for 6 minutes on each side to achieve searing. Push the salmon to the pan's edges for space for the kale after the salmon has been prepared for 12 minutes. Toss the kale inside the pan drippings after adding salt, red pepper, and flakes. The greens should wilt after 3 minutes of cooking under cover. Serve the braised kale and salmon fillets on four dinner plates.

Nutritional Info: Calories: 438 kcal, Protein: 26.3g, Carb: 5.8g, Fat: 33g.

2. Scallops and Mozza Broccoli Mash

(Setup Time: 5 minutes | Cooked in: 35 minutes | How many people: 4 | Difficulty: Easy)

Recipe Components:

Mozza Broccoli Mash:

- 570 g or 6 cups broccoli florets
- 2-in/5-cm 1 piece fresh ginger root, grated
- 70 g or ½ cup mozzarella cheese (regular or dairy-free), shredded
- 55 g or ¼ cup coconut ghee or oil, or 60 ml ¼ cup avocado oil
- 4 minced cloves of garlic
- 160 ml or ⅔ cup chicken bone broth

Scallops:
- ¼ tsp sea salt, finely ground
- 2 tbsp coconut oil, ghee, or avocado oil
- 455 g or 1 pound sea scallops
- ¼ tsp black pepper, ground
- Lemon wedges to serve

Preparation Steps: Making the mash: Warm the oil slowly in a big frying pan. Cook the broccoli, ginger, and garlic for 5 minutes, uncovered, or once the garlic is aromatic. Add the liquid, put the lid, and cook for 25 minutes on low heat, or until the broccoli is easily mashed. Prepare the scallops for around 5 minutes until the broccoli is done: After patting the scallops dry, sprinkle salt and pepper over both sides. The oil is heated in a frying pan of around average size over a moderate flame. Add the scallops to the heated oil. Cook each side for 2 minutes or until lightly browned. Add the cheese and mash using a fork after cooking the broccoli. On top of the scallops, divide the mashed potatoes among 4 dinner plates. Enjoy your meal with lemon wedges!

Nutritional Info: Calories: 353 kcal, Protein: 19.2g, Carb: 12g, Fat: 25.4g.

3. Noodles and glazed Salmon

(Setup Time: 5 minutes | Cooked in: 20 minutes | How many people: 4 | Difficulty: Moderate)

Recipe Components:
- 60 ml or ¼ cup coconut amino
- 2 tbsp apple cider vinegar
- 4 minced cloves of garlic
- 455 g or 1 pound salmon fillets, cut into 4 equal portions
- 2 sliced green onions
- 1 tsp sesame seeds
- 75 ml or ¼ cup plus 2 tbsp avocado oil, divided
- 2 tbsp plus 2 tsps tomato paste

- 2-in/5-cm 1 piece fresh ginger root, grated

- ½ tsp sea salt, finely ground

- 7-oz/198-g 2 packages konjac noodles or the same amount of other low-carb noodles of choice

- Handful of cilantro leaves, fresh and roughly chopped

Preparation Steps: In a large frying pan, flame 2 tbsp of oil over medium heat. Make the sauce once the oil is warming up: Mix the tomato paste, ginger, vinegar, garlic, coconut amino, salt, and the remaining ¼ cup of oil in a small bowl. After adding the salmon to the heated pan, lower the heat and slather it with the sauce. Any leftover sauce should be drizzled immediately into the pan. 15 minutes on low heat, covered, until seared and just barely heated through. When the salmon is finished cooking, pile it up in the pan on one side, leaving room for the noodles. Toss the green onions and noodles in the remaining sauce after adding them to the pan. Then, top the noodles with the cooked salmon. Just enough time to heat your noodles is another three to five minutes of cooking. Salmon should be topped with cilantro and sesame seeds. On four dinner plates, distribute the noodles and salmon, top with any remaining pan sauce, and serve.

Nutritional Info: Calories: 333 kcal, Protein: 24.7g, Carb: 8.2g, Fat: 22.4g.

4. Buttered Salmon

(Setup Time: 10 minutes | Cooked in: 10 minutes | How many people: 2 | Difficulty: Easy)

Recipe Components:

- Salt and black pepper, ground
- 2 salmon fillets
- 1 tbsp. melted butter

Preparation Steps: Place the Cook & Crisp Basket in the Ninja Foodi pot after greasing it. Select Air Crisp and shut the Ninja Foodi with Crisping Lid. For five minutes, set the thermostat to 360 degrees Fahrenheit. To start preheating, press "Start/Stop." After each salmon fillet has been seasoned with salt and pepper, drizzle it with melted butter. Open the cover after preheating. Arrange the salmon fillets in a single layer in the heated Cook & Crisp Basket. Select Air Crisp and shut the Ninja Foodi having Crisping Lid. For 10 minutes, raise the temperature to 360 degrees Fahrenheit. To start cooking, click Start/Stop. Serve warm.

Nutritional Info: Calories: 276 kcal, Protein: 33.1g, Carb: 1g, Fat: 16.3g.

5. Glazed Salmon Fillets

(Setup Time: 10 minutes | Cooked in: 13 minutes | How many people: 2 | Difficulty: Easy)

Recipe Components:

- 2 tbsp bacon syrup
- 2 tsps water
- 3 tbsp soy sauce, low-sodium
- 2 tsps lemon juice, fresh
- 2 salmon fillets

Preparation Steps: In a small bowl, combine all of the ingredients except the salmon. Reserve roughly half of your mixture in a small basin. The remaining mixture is added, and the fish is well coated. For approximately two hours, marinate covered in the refrigerator. In the Ninja Foodi pot, arrange the Cook & Crisp Basket. Select Air Crisp and shut the Ninja Foodi with Crisping Lid. For five minutes, set the thermostat to 355 degrees Fahrenheit. For the preheating to start, press Start/Stop. Open the cover after preheating. Salmon fillets should be added to the Cook & Crisp Basket. Select Air Crisp and shut the Ninja Foodi with Crisping Lid. For 13 minutes, set the thermostat to 355 degrees Fahrenheit. To start cooking, click Start/Stop. Flip all salmon fillets over and brush with the leftover marinade after 8 minutes. Serve warm.

Nutritional Info: Calories: 181 kcal, Protein: 28.2g, Carb: 4g, Fat: 4.7g.

6. Seasoned Catfish

(Setup Time: 15 minutes | Cooked in: 23 minutes | How many people: 4 | Difficulty: Easy)

Recipe Components:

- 2 tbsp Italian seasoning
- 1 tbsp. olive oil
- 4 catfish fillets
- Salt and black pepper, ground
- 1 tbsp. chopped fresh parsley

Preparation Steps: Place the Cook & Crisp Basket inside the Ninja Foodi pot after greasing it. Select Air Crisp and shut the Ninja Foodi with Crisping Lid. For five minutes, set the thermostat to 400 degrees Fahrenheit. For the preheating to start, press Start/Stop. After liberally seasoning all fish fillets with salt, pepper, and seasoning, drizzle oil over them. Open the cover after preheating. The Cook & Crisp Basket should be filled with the catfish fillets. Select Air Crisp and shut the Ninja Foodi with Crisping Lid. For 20 minutes, set the thermostat to 400 degrees Fahrenheit. To start cooking, click Start/Stop. When the fish fillets are halfway done, flip them. Serve hot with parsley as a garnish.

Nutritional Info: Calories: 205 kcal, Protein: 17.7g, Carb: 0.8g, Fat: 14.2g.

7. Parsley Tilapia

(Setup Time: 15 minutes | Cooked in: 1 hour 30 minutes | How many people: 6 | Difficulty: Moderate)

Recipe Components:

- Salt and black pepper, ground
- 3 tsps lemon rind, fresh and grated finely
- 2 tbsp. butter, unsalted and melted
- 6 tilapia fillets
- ½ cup chopped yellow onion
- ¼ cup parsley, freshly chopped

Preparation Steps: Grease the Ninja Foodi pot. Make liberal use of black pepper and salt while seasoning the tilapia fillets. Put the tilapia fillets in the Ninja Foodi pot that has been prepared. Spread the onion, parsley, and lemon rind equally over the fillets before adding the melted butter. Select Slow Cooker, and then close your Ninja Foodi with a crisping cover.

Set for 1 ½ hours on Low. To start cooking, click Start/Stop. Serve warm.

Nutritional Info: Calories: 133 kcal, Protein: 21.3g, Carb: 1.3g, Fat: 4.9g.

8. Cod with Tomatoes

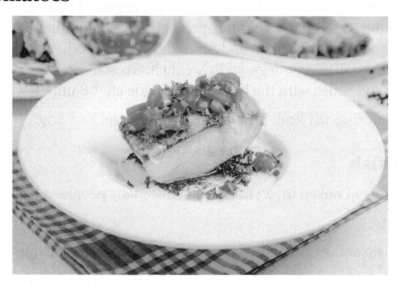

(Setup Time: 15 minutes | Cooked in: 6 minutes | How many people: 4 | Difficulty: Easy)

Recipe Components:

- 2 tbsp rosemary, freshly chopped
- 2 minced garlic cloves
- Salt and black pepper, ground

- 1-pound halved cherry tomatoes
- 4 cod fillets
- 1 tbsp. olive oil

Preparation Steps: Half of the cherry tomatoes and the rosemary should be placed in the base of a big heatproof bowl that has been oiled. Arrange the rest of the tomatoes on top, and then set the fish fillets on top of them. Garlic should be sprinkled on top of the oil. Place the bowl in the Ninja Foodie's bottom. Put the pressure lid on the Ninja Foodi and turn its pressure valve to the Seal position to close it. Select Pressure, then High heat for 6 minutes. To start cooking, click Start/Stop. Change the valve's setting to Vent and perform a quick release. Place the tomatoes and fish fillets on plates for serving. Serve after seasoning with black pepper and salt.

Nutritional Info: Calories: 149 kcal, Protein: 21.4g, Carb: 6g, Fat: 5g.

9. Parmesan Tilapia

(Setup Time: 15 minutes | Cooked in: 4 hours | How many people: 4 | Difficulty: Moderate)

Recipe Components:

- ¼ cup mayonnaise
- Salt and black pepper, ground
- 2 tbsp cilantro, freshly chopped

- ½ cup grated Parmesan cheese
- ¼ cup lemon juice, fresh
- 4 tilapia fillets

Preparation Steps: All ingredients—except the tilapia fillets and cilantro—should be combined in a bowl. Evenly spread the mayonnaise mixture over the fillets. Over a big piece of foil, arrange the filets. To seal the fillets, wrap all foil around them. Place the foil package in the Ninja Foodi's bottom. Select Slow Cooker, and then close your Ninja Foodi with a crisping cover. Set for 3 to 4 hours on low. Press "Start/Stop" to start the stove. Serve hot with cilantro as a garnish.

Nutritional Info: Calories: 223 kcal, Protein: 25.2g, Carb: 0.3g, Fat: 13.5g.

10. Crispy Tilapia

(Setup Time: 15 minutes | Cooked in: 14 minutes | How many people: 4 | Difficulty: Easy)

Recipe Components:

- 1 packet of dry dressing mix, ranch-style
- 2 eggs, organic
- ¾ cup crushed pork rinds
- 2½ tbsp olive oil
- 4 tilapia fillets

Preparation Steps:

1. Place the Cook & Crisp Basket inside the Ninja Foodi pot after greasing it.
2. Select Air Crisp and shut the Ninja Foodi with Crisping Lid. For five minutes, set the thermostat to 355 degrees Fahrenheit. To start preheating, press "Start/Stop."
3. The eggs should be beaten in a small basin. Add the oil, ranch dressing, and pork rinds to another bowl and stir once a crumbly mixture forms.
4. Fish fillets are dipped in egg and then coated with a combination of pig rinds.
5. Take the lid off and let it preheat. Arrange the tilapia fillets in a single layer in the prepared Cook & Crisp Basket.
6. Select Air Crisp and shut the Ninja Foodi with Crisping Lid.
7. For 14 minutes, preheat the oven to 350 degrees Fahrenheit. To start cooking, click Start/Stop. Serve warm.

Nutritional Info: Calories: 304 kcal, Protein: 38g, Carb: 0.4g, Fat: 16.8g.

Chapter 8: Sauces & Dressing Recipes

Below are the recipes.

---

1. Easy & quick barbecue sauce

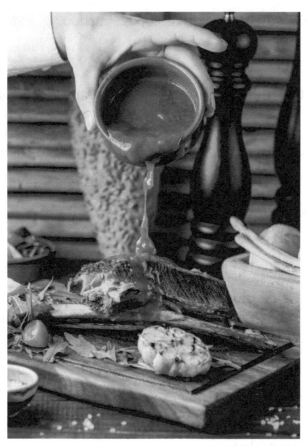

(Setup Time: 5 minutes | Cooked in: 0 minutes | How many people: 1 ¼ cups | Difficulty: Easy)

Recipe Components:

- 80 ml or ⅓ cup (80 ml) water
- 2 tbsp coconut amino
- ½ tsp garlic powder
- ½ tsp paprika
- ¼ tsp black pepper, ground

- 80 ml or ⅓ cup balsamic vinegar
- 6-oz/170-g 1 tin tomato paste
- 1 tbsp. Dijon mustard
- ½ tsp onion powder
- ½ tsp sea salt, finely ground

Preparation Steps: In a 16-ounce (475 ml) or big airtight container, combine all the ingredients. Shake the cover while incorporating.

Nutritional Info: Calories: 11 kcal, Protein: 0.4g, Carb: 2.1g, Fat: 0.1g.

2. Teriyaki sauce and marinade

(Setup Time: 5 minutes | Cooked in: 0 minutes | How many people: 1 ½ cups | Difficulty: Easy)

Recipe Components:

- 60 ml or ¼ cup coconut amino
- 1 tbsp. apple cider vinegar
- 1 tsp ginger powder
- 240 ml or 1 cup of light-tasting oil, such as light olive oil or avocado oil
- 2 tbsp erythritol, confectioners'-style
- 1 tsp garlic powder
- 1 tsp sea salt, finely ground

Preparation Steps: In a 16-ounce (475 ml) or big airtight container, combine all the ingredients. Shake the cover while incorporating. Shake the container slightly before serving and take a bite.

Nutritional Info: Calories: 85 kcal, Protein: 0g, Carb: 0.7g, Fat: 9.1g.

3. Avocado mousse

(Setup Time: 2 minutes | Cooked in: 10 minutes | How many people: 7 | Difficulty: Easy)

Recipe Components:

- 3 tbsp. Erythritol
- 1 tsp. butter
- 1 tsp. of cocoa powder
- 2 avocados, cored and peeled
- 1/3 cup heavy cream
- 1 tsp. vanilla extract

Preparation Steps: For five minutes, preheat the Ninja Foodi in the sauté mode. Meanwhile, puree the avocado and combine it with the erythritol. Melt the butter after adding it to the saucepan. Stir thoroughly after adding the mashed avocado combination. Cocoa powder should be added and mixed well. Three minutes to sauté the ingredients. While doing this, whisk your heavy cream for two minutes at high speed. Place the warm avocado purée in a bowl and chill it in the refrigerator. Add the vanilla extract and heavy cream after the avocado mash has warmed to room temperature. Gently stir to create swirls of white chocolate. Place the mousse in tiny cups and refrigerate for 4 hours.

Nutritional Info: Calories: 144 kcal, Protein: 1.3g, Carb: 10.5g, Fat: 13.9g.

4. Ranch dressing

(Setup Time: 5 minutes | Cooked in: 0 minutes | How many people: 2 cups | Difficulty: Easy)

Recipe Components:

- 120 ml or ½ cup full-fat coconut milk
- 2 tbsp fresh chives, sliced
- 1 tbsp. white onions, minced

- 1 tbsp. apple cider vinegar
- ¼ tsp sea salt, finely ground
- 210 g or 1 cup mayonnaise
- 3 tbsp fresh parsley, finely chopped
- 2 small minced cloves of garlic
- 1 tbsp. fresh dill, finely chopped
- 1 tbsp. lemon juice
- ⅛ tsp black pepper, ground

Preparation Steps: In a 20-ounce (600 ml) or big airtight container, combine all the ingredients. Shake the cover while incorporating. Shake the container slightly before serving and take a bite.

Nutritional Info: Calories: 57 kcal, Protein: 0.1g, Carb: 0.4g, Fat: 6.1g.

5. Thai dressing

(Setup Time: 5 minutes | Cooked in: 0 minutes | How many people: 1 cup | Difficulty: Easy)

Recipe Components:
- 60 ml or ¼ cup full-fat coconut milk
- 2 tbsp coconut amino
- 1 tbsp. lime juice
- ½ tsp cayenne pepper
- 70 g or ¼ cup smooth almond butter, unsweetened
- 2 tbsp apple cider vinegar
- 2 tbsp sesame oil, toasted
- 1 tsp garlic powder
- ½ tsp sea salt, finely ground

Preparation Steps: In a 12-ounce (350 ml) or big airtight container, combine all the ingredients. Shake the cover while incorporating. Shake the container slightly before serving and take a bite. Keep for up to 5 days in the refrigerator.

Nutritional Info: Calories: 22 kcal, Protein: 0.1g, Carb: 0.7g, Fat: 2g.

Chapter 9: Dessert Recipes

Below are the recipes.

1. Raspberry dump cake

(Setup Time: 10 minutes | Cooked in: 30 minutes | How many people: 10 | Difficulty: Easy)

Recipe Components:

- 1 ½ cup coconut flour
- ¼ cup Erythritol
- 1 tbsp. melted butter
- ½ tsp. vanilla extract
- ½ cup raspberries
- 1/3 cup almond milk
- 1 whisked egg
- 1 tsp. baking powder
- 1 tsp. lemon juice

Preparation Steps: Harmonize the dry components. Then, stir in the egg, butter, and almond milk. Lemon juice and vanilla extract are added. Stir your mixture well. Get a liquid batter right away. Put the raspberries in a layer into the silicone mold. Over the raspberries, pour the batter. Put the mold on your rack and put the Ninja Foodi basket over it. Put the air fryer's cover on and choose Bake. The cake should be baked for about 30 minutes at 350°F. After baking, thoroughly refrigerate the cake. Flip over and place on the serving platter.

Nutritional Info: Calories: 107 kcal, Protein: 4.3g, Carb: 15.1g, Fat: 4.5g.

2. Brownie batter

(Setup Time: 5 minutes | Cooked in: 4 minutes | How many people: 5 | Difficulty: Easy)

Recipe Components:

- ¼ cup heavy cream
- 1 tbsp. Erythritol
- 3 tbsp. butter
- 1 oz. dark chocolate
- 1/3 cup almond flour
- 3 tbsp. cocoa powder
- ½ tsp. vanilla extract

Preparation Steps: To create the layer, spread the almond flour in the springform pan. Put the springform pan into the pot afterwards, and close the air fryer cover. The almond flour should be cooked for 3 minutes at 400 degrees F or until brown. Meanwhile, add heavy cream and cocoa powder; whisk all heavy cream until smooth. Add erythritol and vanilla essence. Ninja Foodi's almond flour should be taken out and well chilled. Put the dark chocolate and butter in the saucepan and set the temperature to Sauté for 1 minute. Add the softened butter to your heavy cream mixture. Then, include almond flour and chocolate. Serve the mixture after homogenizing it.

Nutritional Info: Calories: 159 kcal, Protein: 2.5g, Carb: 9g, Fat: 14.9g.

3. Ketone Gummies

(Setup Time: 40 minutes | Cooked in: 5 minutes | How many people: 8 | Difficulty: Easy)

Recipe Components:

- 8 hulled strawberries (frozen and defrosted or fresh)
- 2 tsps exogenous ketones
- 120 ml or ½ cup lemon juice
- 2 tbsp gelatin, unflavored
- Silicone mold having eight 2-tbsp. or bigger cavities

Preparation Steps: Have your preferred silicone mold on hand. To produce 8 gummies, people prefer to utilize a big silicone ice cube tray and scoop 2 tsps of the ingredients into each cavity. If you don't have a silicone mold, use a metal or silicone baking pan that is 8 inches (20 cm) square. Line a metal pan with parchment paper and let it hang over the sides for easy cleanup. Strawberries, gelatin, and lemon juice can be blended or processed until smooth in a food processor or blender. Place the contents of the bowl into the small saucepan and bring to a simmer. Cook for 5 minutes or until the mixture is very liquid. After the flame is switched off, exogenous ketones are introduced. The batter can be poured into a baking dish or divided among the eight wells of a mold. Allow to sit for 30 minutes in the fridge. Cut into 8 squares if utilizing a baking pan.

Nutritional Info: Calories: 19 kcal, Protein: 3.2g, Carb: 1.2g, Fat: 0.2g.

4. Soft-Serve Chocolate Ice Cream

(Setup Time: 55 minutes | Cooked in: 0 minutes | How many people: 4 | Difficulty: Easy)

Recipe Components:

- 40 g or ¼ cup collagen peptides or protein powder (optional)
- 2 tbsp smooth almond butter, unsweetened
- 1 tbsp. erythritol or 3 drops liquid stevia
- 13½-oz/400-ml 1 tin coconut milk, full-fat
- 25 g or ¼ cup unflavored MCT oil powder (optional)
- 2 tbsp cocoa powder
- 1 tsp vanilla extract

Preparation Steps: Combine everything in a blender or food processor. Mix it up until everything is evenly distributed. Place the mixture in the freezer for about 30 minutes after dividing it among 4 freezer-safe serving dishes. Remove from the freezer after 30 minutes and mash using a fork once the ice cream is creamy.

If it's still too fluid and doesn't become soft-serve consistency when you mash it, put it in the freezer for 15 minutes before mashing it with a fork. Enjoy right now.

Nutritional Info: Calories: 419 kcal, Protein: 5.8g, Carb: 9g, Fat: 46.6g.

5. Pumpkin pie

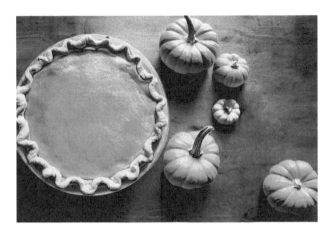

(Setup Time: 10 minutes | Cooked in: 25 minutes | How many people: 6 | Difficulty: Easy)

Recipe Components:

- ¼ cup heavy cream
- 1 tbsp. butter
- 1 tbsp. pumpkin puree
- 1 tsp. Pumpkin spices
- 1 cup coconut flour

- 1 egg, whisked
- 2 tbsp. liquid stevia
- 1 tsp. Apple cider vinegar
- ½ tsp. baking powder

Preparation Steps: Baking powder, liquid stevia, heavy cream, melted butter, and apple cider vinegar should all be combined. Add coconut flour and pumpkin puree. Spices of pumpkin are now added, and the dough is smoothed. Place the Ninja Foodi basket with the batter inside, and then shut the air fryer lid. The "Bake" mode to 360 degrees Fahrenheit. For 25 minutes, bake the pie. Once the allotted time has passed, allow the pie to cool until room temperature.

Nutritional Info: Calories: 127 kcal, Protein: 3.8g, Carb: 14.2g, Fat: 6.6g.

6. Superpower Fat Bombs

(Setup Time: 45 minutes | Cooked in: 0 minutes | How many people: 8 | Difficulty: Easy)

Recipe Components:

- 40 g or ¼ cup collagen peptides or protein powder
- 2 tbsp cocoa powder
- 1 tbsp. cacao nibs
- 1 tbsp. plus 1 tsp confectioners'-style erythritol or 4 drops liquid stevia

- Silicone mold along 8 2-tbsp. or larger cavities (optional)
- 145 g or ⅔ cup cacao butter, coconut oil, or ghee, melted
- 25 g or ¼ cup MCT oil powder, unflavored
- 2 tbsp flax seeds, roughly ground
- 1 tsp instant coffee granules
- Pinch of sea salt, finely ground

Preparation Steps: Have your preferred silicone mold on hand. We prefer to produce 8 cubes using a large silicone ice cube tray and spoon 2 tsps of the ingredients into each well. If you don't have a silicone mold, you can still make a wonderful bark out of this. Line a metal or silicone 8-inch (20-cm) square baking sheet with baking paper, leaving some parchment hanging over the sides for easy removal. All the ingredients should be whisked together in a medium-sized bowl until smooth. Pour the mixture into the baking pan or divide it among the 8 holes in the silicone mold. When using cacao butter, transfer to the refrigerator and set for 15 minutes; when using coconut oil or ghee, let set for 30 minutes. For serving, divide the bark into 8 pieces using a baking sheet. Keep refrigerated for up to 10 days or frozen for up to 2 months in an airtight container. No need to defrost; enjoy directly from the freezer.

Nutritional Info: Calories: 136 kcal, Protein: 5.8g, Carb: 3g, Fat: 12.3g.

7. Blueberry crumbles with cream topping

(Setup Time: 5 minutes | Cooked in: 25 minutes | How many people: 6 | Difficulty: Easy)

Recipe Components:

- 110 g or 1 cup blanched almond flour
- 65 g or ⅓ cup erythritol
- 1 tsp cinnamon, ground
- 510 g or 18 ozs of blueberries, frozen or fresh
- 70 g or ⅓ cup coconut oil or ghee at room temperature
- 2 tbsp coconut flour
- 250 g or 1 cup coconut cream, or 240 ml or 1 cup full-fat coconut milk to serve

Preparation Steps:

Prepare the oven to 350 degrees Fahrenheit (177 degrees C). Put the blueberries in an oven-safe dish that's 8 inches (20 centimeters) square. Combine the almond flour, erythritol, oil, coconut flour, and cinnamon in a bowl and whisk with a fork until the mixture resembles crumbs. Sprinkle the crumble on top of the blueberries. After browning the top requires a further 22–25 minutes in the oven. Rest for ten minutes after removing from oven, then cut into six servings. Dishes, how many? Sprinkle two to three tsps of coconut cream onto each serving.

Nutritional Info: Calories: 388 kcal, Protein: 4.9g, Carb: 12.7g, Fat: 33.4g.

60-Day Meal Plan

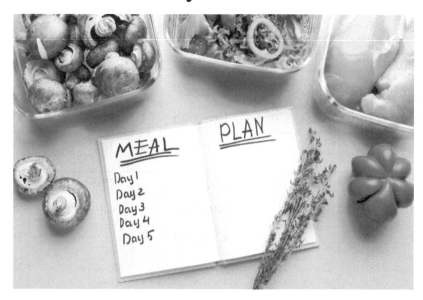

Days	Breakfast	Snack	Lunch	Snack	Dinner
Day 1	Vanilla muffins	Almond Bites	BBQ Chicken	Roasted Marinated mushrooms	Crispy Tilapia
Day 2	Superpower Fat Bombs	Tuna Cucumber Boats	Sriracha carrots	Ginger Cookies	Beef Jerky
Day 3	Mushroom Breaded Nuggets	Vanilla Yogurt	Salmon and Kale	Avocado mousse	Keto-Friendly Chicken Tortillas
Day 4	Vegetable tart	Avocado bacon-wrapped fries	Crispy thighs and mash	Ketone Gummies	Parmesan Tilapia
Day 5	Pumpkin pie	Ginger broccoli soup	Turkey Cutlets	Brownie batter	Bacon Wrapped Beef Tenderloins

Day 6	Liver Bites	Raspberry dump cake	The Premium Red Pork	Stewed cabbage	Cod with Tomatoes
Day 7	Blueberry crumbles with cream topping	Rosemary Toasted Nuts	Scallops and Mozza Broccoli Mash	Roasted veggie mix	Hot Spicy Paprika Chicken
Day 8	Spinach Quiche	Brussels sprouts	Chili Rubbed Chicken	Keto Diet Snack Plate	Crispy Pork with thyme-lemon cauliflower rice
Day 9	Tapenade	Kale salad with spicy lime-tahini dressing	Happy Burrito Bowl Pork	Soft-Serve Chocolate Ice Cream	Cream of Mushroom–Stuffed Chicken
Day 10	Zucchini Pizza	Jicama Crunchy Fries	Seasoned Catfish	Radish chips and pesto	BBQ beef and slaw
Day 11	Vanilla muffins	Almond Bites	BBQ Chicken	Roasted Marinated mushrooms	Crispy Tilapia
Day 12	Superpower Fat Bombs	Tuna Cucumber Boats	Sriracha carrots	Ginger Cookies	Beef Jerky
Day 13	Mushroom Breaded Nuggets	Vanilla Yogurt	Salmon and Kale	Avocado mousse	Keto-Friendly Chicken Tortillas
Day 14	Vegetable tart	Avocado bacon-wrapped fries	Crispy thighs and mash	Ketone Gummies	Parmesan Tilapia

Day 15	Pumpkin pie	Ginger broccoli soup	Turkey Cutlets	Brownie batter	Bacon Wrapped Beef Tenderloins
Day 16	Liver Bites	Raspberry dump cake	The Premium Red Pork	Stewed cabbage	Cod with Tomatoes
Day 17	Blueberry crumbles with cream topping	Rosemary Toasted Nuts	Scallops and Mozza Broccoli Mash	Roasted veggie mix	Hot Spicy Paprika Chicken
Day 18	Spinach Quiche	Brussels sprouts	Chili Rubbed Chicken	Keto Diet Snack Plate	Crispy Pork with thyme-lemon cauliflower rice
Day 19	Tapenade	Kale salad with spicy lime-tahini dressing	Happy Burrito Bowl Pork	Soft-Serve Chocolate Ice Cream	Cream of Mushroom–Stuffed Chicken
Day 20	Zucchini Pizza	Jicama Crunchy Fries	Seasoned Catfish	Radish chips and pesto	BBQ beef and slaw
Day 21	Vanilla muffins	Almond Bites	BBQ Chicken	Roasted Marinated mushrooms	Crispy Tilapia
Day 22	Superpower Fat Bombs	Tuna Cucumber Boats	Sriracha carrots	Ginger Cookies	Beef Jerky

Day 23	Mushroom Breaded Nuggets	Vanilla Yogurt	Salmon and Kale	Avocado mousse	Keto-Friendly Chicken Tortillas
Day 24	Vegetable tart	Avocado bacon-wrapped fries	Crispy thighs and mash	Ketone Gummies	Parmesan Tilapia
Day 25	Pumpkin pie	Ginger broccoli soup	Turkey Cutlets	Brownie batter	Bacon Wrapped Beef Tenderloins
Day 26	Liver Bites	Raspberry dump cake	The Premium Red Pork	Stewed cabbage	Cod with Tomatoes
Day 27	Blueberry crumbles with cream topping	Rosemary Toasted Nuts	Scallops and Mozza Broccoli Mash	Roasted veggie mix	Hot Spicy Paprika Chicken
Day 28	Spinach Quiche	Brussels sprouts	Chili Rubbed Chicken	Keto Diet Snack Plate	Crispy Pork with thyme-lemon cauliflower rice
Day 29	Tapenade	Kale salad with spicy lime-tahini dressing	Happy Burrito Bowl Pork	Soft-Serve Chocolate Ice Cream	Cream of Mushroom–Stuffed Chicken
Day 30	Zucchini Pizza	Jicama Crunchy Fries	Seasoned Catfish	Radish chips and pesto	BBQ beef and slaw

Day 31	Vanilla muffins	Almond Bites	BBQ Chicken	Roasted Marinated mushrooms	Crispy Tilapia
Day 32	Superpower Fat Bombs	Tuna Cucumber Boats	Sriracha carrots	Ginger Cookies	Beef Jerky
Day 33	Mushroom Breaded Nuggets	Vanilla Yogurt	Salmon and Kale	Avocado mousse	Keto-Friendly Chicken Tortillas
Day 34	Vegetable tart	Avocado bacon-wrapped fries	Crispy thighs and mash	Ketone Gummies	Parmesan Tilapia
Day 35	Pumpkin pie	Ginger broccoli soup	Turkey Cutlets	Brownie batter	Bacon Wrapped Beef Tenderloins
Day 36	Liver Bites	Raspberry dump cake	The Premium Red Pork	Stewed cabbage	Cod with Tomatoes
Day 37	Blueberry crumbles with cream topping	Rosemary Toasted Nuts	Scallops and Mozza Broccoli Mash	Roasted veggie mix	Hot Spicy Paprika Chicken
Day 38	Spinach Quiche	Brussels sprouts	Chili Rubbed Chicken	Keto Diet Snack Plate	Crispy Pork with thyme-lemon cauliflower rice

Day 39	Tapenade	Kale salad with spicy lime-tahini dressing	Happy Burrito Bowl Pork	Soft-Serve Chocolate Ice Cream	Cream of Mushroom–Stuffed Chicken
Day 40	Zucchini Pizza	Jicama Crunchy Fries	Seasoned Catfish	Radish chips and pesto	BBQ beef and slaw
Day 41	Vanilla muffins	Almond Bites	BBQ Chicken	Roasted Marinated mushrooms	Crispy Tilapia
Day 42	Superpower Fat Bombs	Tuna Cucumber Boats	Sriracha carrots	Ginger Cookies	Beef Jerky
Day 43	Mushroom Breaded Nuggets	Vanilla Yogurt	Salmon and Kale	Avocado mousse	Keto-Friendly Chicken Tortillas
Day 44	Vegetable tart	Avocado bacon-wrapped fries	Crispy thighs and mash	Ketone Gummies	Parmesan Tilapia
Day 45	Pumpkin pie	Ginger broccoli soup	Turkey Cutlets	Brownie batter	Bacon Wrapped Beef Tenderloins
Day 46	Liver Bites	Raspberry dump cake	The Premium Red Pork	Stewed cabbage	Cod with Tomatoes
Day 47	Blueberry crumbles with cream topping	Rosemary Toasted Nuts	Scallops and Mozza Broccoli Mash	Roasted veggie mix	Hot Spicy Paprika Chicken

Day 48	Spinach Quiche	Brussels sprouts	Chili Rubbed Chicken	Keto Diet Snack Plate	Crispy Pork with thyme-lemon cauliflower rice
Day 49	Tapenade	Kale salad with spicy lime-tahini dressing	Happy Burrito Bowl Pork	Soft-Serve Chocolate Ice Cream	Cream of Mushroom–Stuffed Chicken
Day 50	Zucchini Pizza	Jicama Crunchy Fries	Seasoned Catfish	Radish chips and pesto	BBQ beef and slaw
Day 51	Vanilla muffins	Almond Bites	BBQ Chicken	Roasted Marinated mushrooms	Crispy Tilapia
Day 52	Superpower Fat Bombs	Tuna Cucumber Boats	Sriracha carrots	Ginger Cookies	Beef Jerky
Day 53	Mushroom Breaded Nuggets	Vanilla Yogurt	Salmon and Kale	Avocado mousse	Keto-Friendly Chicken Tortillas
Day 54	Vegetable tart	Avocado bacon-wrapped fries	Crispy thighs and mash	Ketone Gummies	Parmesan Tilapia
Day 55	Pumpkin pie	Ginger broccoli soup	Turkey Cutlets	Brownie batter	Bacon Wrapped Beef Tenderloins

Day 56	Liver Bites	Raspberry dump cake	The Premium Red Pork	Stewed cabbage	Cod with Tomatoes
Day 57	Blueberry crumbles with cream topping	Rosemary Toasted Nuts	Scallops and Mozza Broccoli Mash	Roasted veggie mix	Hot Spicy Paprika Chicken
Day 58	Spinach Quiche	Brussels sprouts	Chili Rubbed Chicken	Keto Diet Snack Plate	Crispy Pork with thyme-lemon cauliflower rice
Day 59	Tapenade	Kale salad with spicy lime-tahini dressing	Happy Burrito Bowl Pork	Soft-Serve Chocolate Ice Cream	Cream of Mushroom–Stuffed Chicken
Day 60	Zucchini Pizza	Jicama Crunchy Fries	Seasoned Catfish	Radish chips and pesto	BBQ beef and slaw

Conclusion

The ketogenic diet facilitates the body's transition into ketosis, where fat becomes the primary energy source instead of carbohydrates. Characterized by low carbohydrate intake and a high-fat content, it shows promise in weight reduction, improved blood sugar control, increased satiety, and reduced cholesterol levels. However, its sustainability may pose challenges, and potential drawbacks include an elevated risk of vitamin deficiencies and a potential impact on athletic performance. Before embarking on any new dietary regimen, it is imperative to consult with a healthcare professional and be mindful of potential food allergies or intolerances. While the ketogenic diet proves effective for weight loss and certain health benefits, it is not universally suitable.

Consulting a healthcare expert, considering nutritional needs, planning meals, monitoring macronutrients, anticipating social situations, and seeking support are essential steps to ensure the diet's reliability and acceptability. Sustainability and environmental impact should also factor into the decision-making process when selecting a diet. Before commencing the ketogenic diet, consultation with a healthcare provider is crucial, as it may not be suitable for everyone. Individuals with specific medical conditions or medications, its restrictive nature, and potential drawbacks, such as a higher risk of vitamin deficiencies, should be taken into account. Seeking advice from a physician or nutritionist is paramount before embarking on any new diet. In this book, we have included a comprehensive grocery list and quick recipes to prepare you for the keto diet. The variety of meals available while following the keto diet is extensive, ranging from appetizers, snacks, side dishes, vegetables, meat, poultry, and fish to sauces and desserts. Enjoying delicious meals while effortlessly losing weight is a unique aspect of the keto diet.

ANTI-INFLAMMATORY DIET FOR BEGINNERS

Introduction

The concept of inflammation refers to the enlargement of a specific area in the body, typically accompanied by pain, redness, and heightened warmth. Such manifestations are common when an injury or illness is present, occurring in various parts of the body. While short-term inflammation is characterized by typical symptoms, prolonged inflammation, known as chronic irritation, is linked to the onset of diseases. The body's inflammatory response is a vital defense mechanism and contributes to disease resistance. Despite its positive role in the body's healing process, there are individuals with medical conditions compromising their immune systems, leading to prolonged or chronic inflammation. Chronic inflammation can arise from infections or conditions like psoriasis, asthma, and rheumatoid arthritis. Research suggests a potential link between persistent inflammation and cancer development. Additionally, emerging medical evidence suggests that dietary choices may influence continuous inflammation. Therefore, modifying your diet can be beneficial if you are dealing with inflammation.

Symptoms of inflammation

Several indicators may suggest the presence of inflammation in the body, such as:

- Abdominal bloating
- Joint discomfort
- Appetite loss
- Acid reflux
- Nausea
- Digestive issues (diarrhea, gas, cramping)

If you experience these symptoms, consulting your primary care physician promptly is crucial. They can help determine whether the symptoms align with inflammation or indicate another condition. Fortunately, making simple dietary adjustments can naturally reduce inflammation levels, emphasizing gradual progress towards long-term health. Following an anti-inflammatory diet is a method that promotes consistent improvement for overall well-being.

CHAPTER 1: Decoding the Essence of the "Anti-Inflammatory Diet"

1.1 Grasping the Nature of Persistent Inflammation

Inflammation serves as a fundamental and inherent aspect of the body's defense mechanism, acting as a response to injuries, infections, and various threats. While acute inflammation is a brief and beneficial reaction aiding in healing, prolonged inflammation can lead to chronic inflammatory conditions associated with diverse health challenges.

Inflammatory Afflictions and Well-being

Numerous diseases and ailments are closely linked to chronic inflammation, encompassing arthritis, cardiovascular ailments, diabetes, and autoimmune disorders. Understanding these correlations is pivotal for the effective management and prevention of health issues. Autoimmune conditions like rheumatoid arthritis and lupus involve the immune system erroneously attacking healthy tissues, resulting in persistent inflammation. The involvement of chronic inflammation in the formation of arterial plaques elevates the risk of cardiovascular events like heart attacks and strokes. Additionally, neurodegenerative conditions such as Alzheimer's exhibit connections to chronic inflammation. Cutting-edge scientific research indicates the significant impact of diet on either fostering or mitigating chronic inflammation. Certain foods possess anti-inflammatory properties, with diets rich in antioxidants, polyphenols, and omega-3 fatty acids exhibiting inflammation-reducing effects. Beyond diet, lifestyle choices wield considerable influence in either aggravating or alleviating inflammation. It is crucial to comprehend how daily decisions can sway your inflammatory status and overall health.

- **Exercise and Inflammation:** Substantial evidence supports the anti-inflammatory benefits of exercise on the body.

- **Stress Management:** Chronic stress can trigger the release of stress hormones that fuel inflammation.

- **Sleep Quality:** Disrupted sleep patterns and sleep disorders can contribute to chronic inflammation.

- **Smoking and Alcohol Consumption:** Both smoking and excessive alcohol consumption are recognized exacerbators of inflammation

Inflammation's Nexus with Chronic Ailments

Chronic inflammation is progressively acknowledged as a common denominator linking numerous chronic diseases. By recognizing the profound impact of inflammation on these enduring illnesses, one gains the insight needed to make informed decisions that foster not only a life free from chronic inflammation but also enduring health and well-being.

- **Cardiovascular Health:** Persistent inflammation significantly contributes to atherosclerosis, the accrual of plaque in the arteries.

- **Autoimmune Diseases:** Conditions like rheumatoid arthritis, lupus, and multiple sclerosis are characterized by persistent inflammation.

- **Cancer and Inflammation:** Evolving evidence suggests that continual inflammation may contribute to the development of cancer.

- **Metabolic Conditions:** Chronic inflammation is intricately linked to conditions such as diabetes and obesity.

1.2 Inflammation-Reducing Dietary Approaches

Indeed, there is no singular diet that assures the reduction of inflammation for specific health conditions, arthritis being no exception. Various diets aim to alleviate inflammation, such as the Dietary Pattern and Dr. Weil's recommended diet. Both emphasize the consumption of foods influencing body irritation or contributing to its relief. Diets tailored to diminish inflammation naturally incorporate products known for their anti-inflammatory properties, discouraging the intake of foods provoking inflammatory responses. Consuming antioxidant-rich foods is pivotal for an anti-inflammatory diet, as antioxidants combat free radicals, preventing potential cell damage and subsequent inflammation. Numerous studies have highlighted the ability of plant-based antioxidants to counteract the harmful effects of free radicals, which, when accumulated, can harm the body's cells. Consequently, inflammation-reducing diets focus on internal cleansing and overall body maintenance, enhancing the immune system and digestion with regular adherence.

Prominent Anti-Inflammatory Dietary Approaches

Several diets have gained acclaim for their potential to alleviate inflammation and enhance overall well-being. These diets center around whole, nutrient-dense foods, effectively reducing pro-inflammatory elements. Notable anti-inflammatory diets include:

- **Mediterranean Diet:** Centered on fruits, vegetables, whole grains, olive oil, lean meats, and a modest amount of red wine, this diet boasts anti-inflammatory benefits due to its high antioxidant and omega-3 fatty acid content.

- **DASH Diet (Dietary Approaches to Stop Hypertension):** Comprising fruits, vegetables, healthy grains, lean meats, and low-fat dairy, the DASH diet, developed to control hypertension, proves potent in combating inflammation with its nutrient-dense components.

- **Anti-Inflammatory Diet by Dr. Weil:** Dr. Andrew Weil's recommended diet incorporates anti-inflammatory foods like dark leafy greens, berries, fatty fish, and spices such as turmeric. It discourages inflammatory options like processed meals and sweets.

Selecting an Inflammation-Alleviating Diet

Numerous recognized dietary regimens, including the Mediterranean Diet, DASH Diet, and Dr. Weil's Anti-Inflammatory Diet, effectively reduce inflammation. Subsequent chapters will delve into these diverse dietary plans. Opting for the right inflammation-reducing diet involves considering personal preferences, dietary constraints, and health objectives. Whether embracing the Mediterranean diet, DASH diet, or a personalized approach, the fundamental principles endure: prioritize unprocessed, whole foods, minimize or eliminate processed sugars and unhealthy fats, and emphasize nutrient-dense choices. Success lies in adopting a diet that can be consistently maintained—a commitment to sustainable, positive changes in dietary habits rather than rigid rules.

1.3 Different Anti-Inflammatory Food Choices

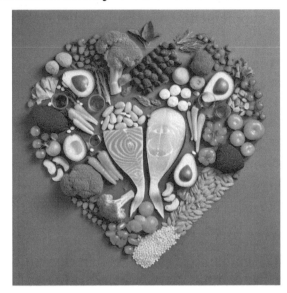

Certain foods stand out for their exceptional ability to combat inflammation, often due to their richness in antioxidants, omega-3 fatty acids, and other inflammation-soothing nutrients. Key anti-inflammatory foods include:

- **Fatty Fish:** Rich in omega-3 fatty acids, fish like salmon, mackerel, sardines, and trout have demonstrated inflammation-reducing properties.

- **Leafy Greens:** Vegetables such as spinach, kale, and collard greens are prime examples of anti-inflammatory choices.

- **Berries:** Blueberries, strawberries, and raspberries, abundant in antioxidants called flavonoids, exhibit powerful anti-inflammatory effects.

- **Nuts and Seeds:** Almonds, walnuts, flaxseeds, and chia seeds, packed with beneficial nutrients, contribute to an anti-inflammatory diet.

- **Turmeric:** This spice boasts curcumin, a compound renowned for robust anti-inflammatory and antioxidant characteristics.

Supplements and Natural Remedies

In the pursuit of inflammation management and overall well-being, dietary modifications represent just one facet. Supplements and natural remedies complement these efforts, enhancing the body's inflammation-handling capacity, reinforcing the immune system, and fostering a more vibrant life:

- **Omega-3 Fatty Acids:** Abundant in fatty fish, omega-3 fatty acids like eicosapentaenoic acid (EPA) and docosahexaenoic acid (DHA) possess scientifically validated anti-inflammatory effects. Incorporating omega-3-rich foods or high-quality fish oil supplements aids in inflammation reduction.

- **Turmeric and Curcumin:** Curcumin, an active compound in turmeric, functions as a potent antioxidant and anti-inflammatory agent. Consuming raw turmeric, cooking with it, or taking curcumin capsules provides health benefits.

- **Ginger:** With anti-inflammatory potential, ginger contains gingerol, a bioactive compound alleviating inflammation and pain. It can be integrated into the diet, used in ginger tea, or taken as supplements, especially beneficial for digestive issues related to inflammation.

- **Probiotics for Gut Health:** Probiotics, beneficial microorganisms supporting a healthy gut, play a pivotal role in regulating inflammation and enhancing the immune system. Fermented foods like yogurt, kefir, sauerkraut, and dietary supplements are rich sources of probiotics.

- **Boswellia Serrata:** Utilized in traditional medicine, Boswellia serrata (Indian frankincense) and its anti-inflammatory component, boswellic acids, offer potential benefits for conditions like osteoarthritis and inflammatory bowel disease.

Natural Anti-Inflammatories in Your Pantry

Common spices and herbs like cinnamon, rosemary, and green tea possess antioxidants and bioactive compounds, aiding in inflammation reduction. Incorporating these into cooking or enjoying them as herbal teas supports anti-inflammatory efforts.

The Role of Vitamin D

Crucial for immune system health and inflammation control, vitamin D levels can be naturally elevated through outdoor sunlight exposure. Vitamin D supplements may be beneficial, especially in limited sun exposure situations or during the winter months.

Lifestyle Factors that Impact Inflammation

Regular physical activity, effective stress management, and quality sleep form integral parts of an anti-inflammatory lifestyle. Including these practices in daily routines maximizes the effectiveness of anti-inflammatory efforts. Consulting with a healthcare professional or qualified nutritionist is crucial when exploring supplements and natural remedies to ensure alignment with specific needs and circumstances. The synergy between dietary adjustments, supplements, and lifestyle changes contributes to a balanced approach promoting long-term health and vitality.

1.5 Foods that are known to trigger inflammation

Inflammation can result from both dietary habits and consumed items, setting the stage for an anti-inflammatory journey by steering clear of inflammation-inducing foods. This approach serves as a foundational step in initiating change.

These foods fall into six distinct categories:

- Vegetable Oils (Includes Seed Oils)
- High Fructose and Sugary Foods
- Excessive Alcohol
- Artificial Trans Fats
- Refined Carbs
- Processed Meat

Vegetable Oils (Includes Seed Oils). Abundant in omega-6 oils, these oils, while necessary, can contribute to increased inflammation if the omega-6 to omega-3 ratio is skewed. The 20th-century surge in vegetable oil consumption is linked to a rise in inflammatory-related health issues, as per experts. These oils, prevalent in cooking and various processed meals, warrant moderation to prevent or mitigate inflammation.

High Fructose and Sugary Foods. Glucose-rich and high-fructose foods, notably high fructose corn syrup and regular sugar, are primary culprits in daily diets worldwide. Research indicates significant harm from added sugars, impacting the body adversely. While naturally occurring sugars are beneficial, excess intake, such as consuming three sodas daily, correlates with health risks like breast cancer and compromising omega-3 fatty acids' anti-inflammatory effects.

Excess Alcohol. While moderate alcohol consumption may have health benefits, excessive intake can lead to health issues, including inflammation. Conditions like irritable bowel syndrome can emerge, causing the body to accumulate bacterial toxins, potentially harming organs and inducing widespread inflammation.

Artificial Trans Fats. Considered the unhealthiest fats, artificial trans fats result from partial hydrogenation, making unsaturated fats more solid and lessening HDL cholesterol. These fats, present in pastries, cookies, margarine, and fast food, harm endothelial cells and increase heart disease risk. Vigilance in avoiding such fats is crucial for overall health.

Refined Carbs. Distinguishing between beneficial and unnecessary carbohydrates is essential. Refined carbs lack the fiber and vital nutrients present in unprocessed forms, potentially causing inflammation despite an extended shelf life. Fiber regulates blood sugar, promotes satiety, and nourishes beneficial gut bacteria, contributing to overall health.

Processed Meat. Delicious yet linked to health risks, processed meats like jerky, ham, and sausages are associated with stomach cancer, colon cancer, heart disease, and diabetes. Their high concentration of advanced glycation end products (AGEs), formed during cooking, is believed to induce inflammation, with colon cancer development being a notable concern. AGEs are considered a significant contributor to inflammation throughout the body, emphasizing the potential health risks associated with processed meat consumption.

CHAPTER 2: Case Studies and Testimonials

Within this chapter, we delve into authentic narratives of individuals under my care who have embraced the anti-inflammatory diet and lifestyle, yielding remarkable results. These case studies and endorsements offer illuminating perspectives on the transformative effects of an anti-inflammatory approach on overall health and well-being. Each individual has graciously shared their experiences, aiming to inspire and guide you on your path to enhanced health through anti-inflammatory practices.

Sarah's Progression to Arthritis Alleviation. Sarah, a 45-year-old educator, confronted rheumatoid arthritis for over a decade, enduring chronic pain, joint swelling, and fatigue. Traditional treatments fell short, propelling Sarah to explore an anti-inflammatory diet rich in fruits, vegetables, fatty fish, and spices. With added exercise and stress management, Sarah witnessed a substantial reduction in joint pain, heightened energy levels, and regained enjoyment of past activities. Collaborating with her healthcare provider, Sarah successfully decreased reliance on medication, showcasing the potency of lifestyle changes in chronic inflammation management.

John's Endeavor for Heart Health. John, a 52-year-old executive with a family history of cardiac issues, prioritized preventive measures. Embracing the Mediterranean diet, rich in vegetables and fruits while low in saturated fat, John coupled dietary adjustments with regular exercise, stress reduction, and omega-3 fish oil supplementation. Over time, John experienced a significant drop in cholesterol and blood pressure, reducing cardiac risk factors and elevating vitality. His journey exemplifies the positive impact an anti-inflammatory diet can have on cardiovascular health.

Emily's Struggle with Digestive Distress. Emily, a 30-year-old designer, grappled with persistent digestive issues, including bloating and discomfort. Traditional approaches yielded little relief. Exploring a diet featuring probiotics, fiber, and anti-inflammatory foods, Emily incorporated yogurt, kefir, and removed processed foods. Her improved gut health resulted in diminished digestive symptoms, emphasizing the vital role of gut health in inflammation and overall well-being.

James' Triumph over Metabolic Challenges. James, a 58-year-old retiree battling obesity and type 2 diabetes, adopted an anti-inflammatory diet emphasizing whole foods and minimal sugar. Coupled with regular exercise and stress reduction, James witnessed weight loss and stabilized blood sugar levels. Guided by healthcare professionals, he successfully reduced reliance on diabetes medication, showcasing the transformative impact of lifestyle changes on metabolic health.

Maria's Battle with Skin Conditions. Maria, a 35-year-old marketing manager, battled eczema and psoriasis, impacting her confidence. Exploring an anti-inflammatory diet rich in omega-3 fatty acids and antioxidants, she eliminated dairy and processed foods. Over months, Maria observed a significant improvement in her skin, underscoring the link between diet and skin health.

David's Confrontation with Chronic Fatigue. David, a 40-year-old IT specialist, grappled with chronic fatigue syndrome. Conventional treatments offered minimal relief. Adopting a diet low in inflammatory elements and high in nutrient-dense foods, coupled with exercise and improved sleep, David experienced gradual improvements in energy levels and cognitive function, managing chronic fatigue more effectively.

Lisa's Victory Over Allergies. Lisa, a 28-year-old graphic designer, addressed lifelong seasonal allergies through an anti-inflammatory diet rich in quercetin and local honey. Over a year, her allergy symptoms became more manageable, showcasing the potential of an anti-inflammatory diet in allergy management.

These cases underscore the diverse ways individuals have harnessed the benefits of an anti-inflammatory diet to enhance their health. While these stories are inspiring, it's crucial to recognize that every journey is unique. When embarking on your health and wellness through anti-inflammatory practices, consulting with healthcare professionals or certified nutritionists is essential.

2.1 Answers to Common Questions

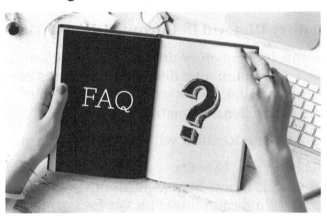

In this section, we will address common inquiries and apprehensions that individuals frequently encounter as they embark on the journey of embracing an anti-inflammatory diet and lifestyle. It's natural to seek clarity along the way, and our aim is to offer lucid and informative answers to assist you in navigating this transformative path to enhanced health.

1 What Exactly Is an Anti-Inflammatory Diet?

The objective of an anti-inflammatory diet is to diminish systemic inflammation by elevating the intake of nutrient-dense foods with recognized anti-inflammatory properties. Staples of the Mediterranean diet, such as fruits, vegetables, whole grains, lean meats, and healthy fats like olive oil and fatty fish, are emphasized. The inflammatory effects of processed meals, added sugars, and artificial trans fats are also minimized or eradicated.

2 Can an Anti-Inflammatory Diet Aid in Weight Loss?

Research indicates that a diet low in inflammatory foods contributes to weight loss. By prioritizing nutrient-dense meals and reducing processed and high-calorie items, this diet promotes satiety through high-fiber and protein-rich foods, potentially leading to reduced overall calorie intake.

3 Are There Specific Foods That Trigger Inflammation?

As we've established, there are a number of foods that are known to cause inflammation. Among these are:

➢ Consuming an excessive amount of sugary meals and drinks, especially those containing high-fructose corn syrup, has been linked to increased inflammation.

> Avoid artificial trans fats, which may be found in many convenience and fast food items but have been linked to inflammation.

> White bread, sugary cereals, and other foods high in refined carbs are linked to insulin surges and inflammation.

> Bacon, sausages, and deli meats are examples of processed meats. The chemicals and preservatives used in these products may promote inflammation.

4 Is an Anti-Inflammatory Diet Suitable for Everyone?

While many can benefit from an anti-inflammatory diet, individual considerations vary. Incorporating this approach necessitates a thoughtful assessment of one's current health, existing food sensitivities, and dietary preferences. For those with pre-existing conditions or special dietary needs, consultation with a healthcare provider or qualified dietitian is advised.

5 Can an Anti-Inflammatory Diet Aid in Chronic Disease Management?

Evidence suggests that an anti-inflammatory diet can contribute to managing chronic illnesses like heart disease, diabetes, and autoimmune disorders. The diet's effectiveness lies in its ability to mitigate systemic inflammation. However, ongoing collaboration with healthcare professionals is crucial for a comprehensive treatment plan.

6 How Long Does It Take to See Results with an Anti-Inflammatory Diet?

The timeline for experiencing the benefits varies among individuals. Some may notice improvements within weeks, while others may require consistent adherence for several months. Emphasizing long-term progress and commitment is key for lasting results.

7 Are Supplements Necessary on an Anti-Inflammatory Diet?

Including more anti-inflammatory foods in the diet can promote regular bowel movements and a healthy gut flora. Conditions like irritable bowel syndrome (IBS) and inflammatory bowel disease (IBD) may benefit from such dietary adjustments.

8 Can an Anti-Inflammatory Diet Enhance Digestive Health?

Including more anti-inflammatory foods in your diet may help your digestive system. This diet can encourage regular bowel movements and healthy gut flora by placing emphasis on fiber-rich foods, including fruits, vegetables, and whole grains. Irritable bowel syndrome (IBS) and inflammatory bowel disease (IBD) are two more illnesses that may benefit from this.

9 Is an Anti-Inflammatory Diet Safe for Pregnant or Breastfeeding Women?

An anti-inflammatory diet can be safe for pregnant and breastfeeding women when appropriately balanced and tailored to their nutritional needs. It can provide essential nutrients and support overall health during this crucial time. However, pregnant and nursing women must talk to their doctor or a qualified nutritionist to determine their individual nutritional needs.

10 Can an Anti-Inflammatory Diet Impact Mental Health?

While more research is needed, there's emerging evidence linking diet, inflammation, and mental health. Nutrient-dense foods can potentially support brain health and mood regulation. Professional mental health treatment, however, should not be replaced when necessary.

11 Are There Any Potential Side Effects of an Anti-Inflammatory Diet?

Considered safe for most individuals due to its emphasis on nutrient-dense foods, an anti-inflammatory diet may cause temporary GI distress in some. Gradual dietary changes and sufficient water intake can mitigate these effects. Those with specific health concerns should consult with a healthcare professional.

12 What Are Some Practical Tips for Staying on Track with an Anti-Inflammatory Diet?

A few simple tricks can make sticking to an anti-inflammatory diet much easier:

➢ Make anti-inflammatory nutrients easily accessible by planning ahead for your meals.

➢ When going grocery shopping, make a list of the foods you need and stick to them so you don't end up with any unnecessary or potentially inflammatory things.

➢ When you cook at home, you get to decide what goes into your meals and how they're prepared.

➢ Keep a food journal to see how your diet influences your health.

➢ Finding a diet buddy or joining a support group can help keep you on track and ensure that you don't give up.

Keep in mind that you don't need to make drastic adjustments all at once in order to get positive results from your anti-inflammatory efforts.

13 Can I Cheat Occasionally on an Anti-Inflammatory Diet?

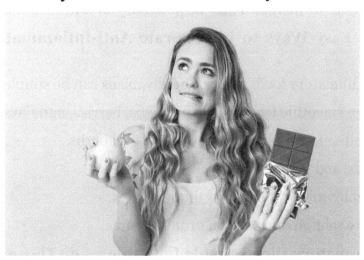

Occasional indulgences or "cheat" meals can be part of a balanced approach to an anti-inflammatory diet. It's essential to strike a balance between enjoying your favorite treats and maintaining the overall principles of the diet. It's important to keep in mind that the key to success is consistency, so don't let the occasional slip up undermine your efforts to lead a healthier lifestyle.

14 Is There a Difference Between an Anti-Inflammatory Diet and Other Diets?

An anti-inflammatory diet differs in some ways from conventional diets. Although there may be some overlap between anti-inflammatory diets and other diets that place an emphasis on full, nutrient-dense foods, the main goal of an anti-inflammatory diet is to decrease inflammation throughout the body.

Those with anti-inflammatory characteristics are promoted, whereas those with the opposite effect are discouraged.

15 How Does Stress Affect Inflammation, and How Can I Manage It?

Chronic stress can elevate cortisol levels, promoting inflammation. Incorporating relaxation techniques, mindfulness, exercise, and adequate sleep into an anti-inflammatory lifestyle is vital for overall well-being.

16 Can an Anti-Inflammatory Diet Benefit Children and Adolescents?

Yes, an anti-inflammatory diet can improve the health of children and teenagers as a whole and cut their chance of developing chronic conditions. Providing them with a diet rich in healthy foods, fruits, vegetables, and lean proteins can aid in their development and growth. However, it's important to talk to a paediatrician or nutritionist about tailoring the diet to their specific needs.

17 What Are Some Common Misconceptions About Anti-Inflammatory Diets?

Misconceptions include the belief that these diets are overly restrictive or that results are immediate. In reality, anti-inflammatory diets can be flexible and require long-term consistency for sustainable improvements.

18 Can I Combine an Anti-Inflammatory Diet with Other Therapies or Medications?

Yes, an anti-inflammatory diet can complement other therapies and medications prescribed by your healthcare provider. It's crucial to inform your healthcare team about dietary changes, as adjustments to medications or therapies may be necessary as your health improves.

19 What Are Some Easy Ways to Incorporate Anti-Inflammatory Foods into My Daily Meals?

Incorporating anti-inflammatory foods into your daily meals can be simple:

➢ Start your day with a smoothie featuring leafy greens, berries, and flaxseeds.

➢ Instead of butter and salt, try cooking with olive oil and herbs.

➢ Snack on nuts, seeds, and fresh fruit.

➢ Add colorful vegetables to your lunch and dinner plates.

➢ Choose fatty fish like salmon or trout as a protein source.

20 Is an Anti-Inflammatory Diet Suitable for Athletes or Those with High Physical Activity Levels?

Yes, an anti-inflammatory diet can be suitable for athletes and individuals with high physical activity levels. It provides essential nutrients for energy, muscle recovery, and overall performance. Adjusting portion sizes and nutrient timing to meet increased energy needs is crucial, and consulting with a sports dietitian can provide personalized guidance.

CHAPTER 3: Anti-inflammatory Breakfast Recipes

3.1 Chia Seed and Milk Pudding

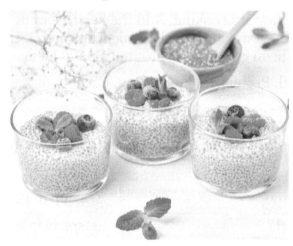

Setup Time: 5 Minutes **Cooked in:** 0 Minutes **How many people:** 6 Persons

Recipe Components:

- 1 cup mixed berries (fresh, for garnishing)
- 4 cups coconut milk (full-fat)
- 3/4 cup coconut yogurt (for topping)
- 1/4 cup coconut chips (toasted for garnishing)
- 1/2 tsp cinnamon (ground)
- 1/2 cup chia seeds
- 3 tbsp honey
- 1 tsp vanilla extract
- 1 tsp turmeric (ground)
- 1/2 tsp ginger (ground)

Preparation Steps: Ginger, turmeric, and cinnamon, together with honey, vanilla extract, and coconut milk, should be combined in a mixing dish. To get a yellowish color, continue to thoroughly combine the ingredients. Put the chia seeds in the bowl and mix everything together. Combine them thoroughly. For around five minutes, you should refrain from stirring the mixture. After the first 5 minutes have passed, give the mixture another stir. Cover the ingredients together. Place it in the refrigerator, where it will stay for at least 6 hours, preferably overnight. The pudding-like consistency will be achieved as a result of the chia seeds expanding and becoming plumper. Distribute the pudding among the four glasses. Put some coconut yogurt, coconut chips, and a combination of berries on top of each glass of pudding. Serve.

Nutrition Calories: 200 Kcal, Proteins: 12g, Fat: 8g, Carbohydrates: 21g

3.2 Scrambled Eggs with Turmeric
Setup Time: 6 Minutes **Cooked in:** 0 Minutes **How many people:** 1 Person

Recipe Components:

- 2 radishes (grated)
- 2 kale leaves (shredded)
- 2 eggs (pastured)
- 1 tbsp. turmeric

- 2 tbsp coconut oil
- 1 small clove of garlic (minced)
- clover and radish sprouts (for topping)
- 1 pinch of cayenne pepper

Preparation Steps: Put some coconut oil in a pan and keep the temperature at medium. Cook the garlic in the skillet. The eggs should be broken up into the pan. Make the eggs into scrambled form by stirring them while they are cooking. Add the kale, cayenne pepper, and turmeric to the scrambled eggs just before they are completely cooked through. Stir. Place on a plate after the transfer. Radishes that have been grated and sprouted should be used as a topping. Serve.

Nutrition Calories: 401 Kcal, Proteins: 25g, Fat: 19g, Carbohydrates: 31g

3.3 Protein-Rich Turmeric Donuts
Setup Time: 5 Minutes **Cooked in:** 10 Minutes **How many people:** 1 Person

Recipe Components:

- 1 1/2 cups cashews (raw)
- 7 Medjool dates (pitted)
- 1/4 cup coconut (shredded)
- 1 tbsp. vanilla protein powder
- 1/4 cup dark chocolate (for topping)
- 2 tsps maple syrup
- 1/4 tsp vanilla essence
- 1 tsp turmeric powder

Preparation Steps: Except for the dark chocolate, place all of the ingredients in a food processor and pulse until smooth. Blend at the highest speed until the mixture forms a dough that is silky, smooth and sticky. Form the dough into a total of eight balls. Donuts should be made by pressing each ball tightly into a mold. Wrap the mold with a cover. Donuts will need to be chilled in the refrigerator for around half an hour. Put one cup of water into a pot and set it to cook over medium heat. Start the water boiling in a pot. Put the dark chocolate in a smaller pot and start heating it up. Put the smaller pan on the upper edge of the larger one that contains the water that is boiling. Chocolate should be stirred until it is completely melted. Remove the doughnuts from the freezer and place them on a plate. Use the melted chocolate to create a glaze for the doughnuts. Serve.

Nutrition Calories: 323 Kcal, Proteins: 29g, Fat: 17g, Carbohydrates: 35g

3.4 Cranberry and Sweet Potato Bars
Setup Time: 6 Minutes **Cooked in:** 10 Minutes **How many people:** 1 Person

Recipe Components:

- 1 cup almond meal
- 1 1/2 cups sweet potato purée
- 1 cup cranberries (fresh)
- 1/3 cup coconut flour
- 1/4 cup water
- 2 eggs
- 2 tbsp coconut oil (melted)
- 2 tbsp maple syrup
- 1 1/2 tsp baking soda

Preparation Steps: Start by preparing the oven to a temperature of 350 degrees F. Combine the eggs, water, melted coconut oil, maple syrup, and sweet potato puree in a large bowl and whisk until smooth. Blend them together well. Sift the almond meal, coconut flour, and baking soda together in a separate mixing bowl. Mix everything up thoroughly.

Mix the two dry components together before adding them to the liquid. The batter must be well mixed. Grease a square baking dish that is 9 inches on a side. Also, cover the interior with parchment paper. The batter should be spread out on the prepared pan. Apply a thin layer of batter to the pan and spread it out evenly with a damp spatula. Put one berry at a time on top of a batter and press down gently. Put it in the oven and bake for 35 minutes, checking it halfway through. When it's totally cold, cut it into 16 pieces.

Nutrition Calories: 130 Kcal, Proteins: 10g, Fat: 5g, Carbohydrates: 11g

3.5 Nutty Choco-Nana Pancakes

Setup Time: 5 Minutes **Cooked in:** 0 Minutes **How many people:** 2 Persons

Recipe Components:

Pancakes:

- 2 eggs (large)
- 2 bananas (ripe)
- 2 tbsp creamy almond butter
- 1/8 tsp salt
- 2 tbsp cacao powder (raw)
- Coconut oil (for greasing)
- 1 tsp pure vanilla extract

Sauce:

- 1/4 cup coconut oil
- 4 tbsp cacao powder (raw)

Preparation Steps: Pancakes: Get a pan ready on low heat. Grease the pan with 1 tbsp. of coconut oil. Put everything you need to make pancakes into a food processor. Pulse all of the ingredients well on high until you get a smooth batter. For each pancake, you'll need about a quarter cup of the batter poured onto the heated griddle. Flip each pancake after 5 minutes of cooking. Turn the pancake over very gently. For a further 2 minutes, flip the meat. Repeat this process until no more batter is available. Sauce may be served alongside or on the pancakes. **Sauce:** Coconut oil, when heated, has a wide range of uses. To the oil, add the cacao powder and mix thoroughly. Get out of the sun. Leave aside.

Nutrition Calories: 621 Kcal, Proteins: 22.4g, Fat: 32g, Carbohydrates: 66g

3.6 Blueberry Avocado Chocolate Muffins

Setup Time: 15 Minutes **Cooked in:** 0 Minutes **How many people:** 2 Persons

Recipe Components:

- 1/2 cup almond milk (unsweetened)
- 1 cup almond flour
- 1/3 cup coconut sugar
- 1/4 cup cacao powder + 1 tbsp. (raw)
- 1/4 cup blueberries (fresh)
- 2 large eggs (room temperature)
- 1 small avocado (ripe)
- 1/4 tsp salt
- 2 tbsp coconut flour
- 2 tsps baking powder
- 2 tbsp dark chocolate chips

Preparation Steps: Bake at 375 degrees Fahrenheit, which requires preheating the oven. Put paper muffin cups in a muffin tray. Put the eggs, salt, avocados, sugar, and 1 tbsp of cacao powder in a blender and mix until smooth.

The texture should resemble smooth pudding after being blended on high. Mix all the ingredients together in a large bowl. In a large bowl, sift together the cocoa powder, baking soda, almond flour, and coconut flour. Mix everything up thoroughly. Add the almond milk to the mashed avocado and mix well. Toss the flour and salt together in a separate bowl, then add it to the avocado mixture while still whisking. Don't overwork the mixture. The blueberries and chocolate chips should be mixed in. Distribute the batter evenly among the 9 muffin cups. Cook for about 18 minutes at 400 degrees. Do not eat the muffins too warm.

Nutrition Calories: 130 Kcal, Proteins: 10.4g, Fat: 5g, Carbohydrates: 11g

3.7 Tropical Smoothie Bowl

Setup Time: 15 Minutes **Cooked in:** 0 Minutes **How many people:** 2 Persons

Recipe Components:

- 1 cup orange juice
- 1 cup pineapple (frozen)
- 1 cup mango (frozen)
- 1/2 banana
- 1 spoonful of chia
- 1/8 tsp turmeric

Toppings:

- Kiwis (sliced)
- Coconut flakes
- Almonds (chopped)
- Strawberries (sliced)

Preparation Steps: Put all the ingredients into a blender and blend them until form a smooth cream. If the mixture is excessively thick, adding a few drops of oranges at a time can do the trick. Split the smoothie in half and serve it in separate bowls. Blend the ingredients together and serve in individual bowls. Serve.

Nutrition Calories: 230 Kcal, Proteins: 11.4g, Fat: 5g, Carbohydrates: 35g

3.8 Smoked Salmon in Scrambled Eggs

Setup Time: 10 Minutes **Cooked in:** 0 Minutes **How many people:** 1 Person

Recipe Components:

- 4 eggs
- 4 slices of smoked salmon (chopped)
- 3 stems of fresh chives (finely chopped)
- Pinch of sea salt
- 2 tbsp coconut milk
- Pinch of black pepper (freshly ground)
- Cooking fat

Preparation Steps: In a large dish, mix together the coconut milk, chives, and eggs. Whisk them together. Season with salt and pepper. Scramble the eggs in a pan with plenty of fat over low to medium heat. Put the eggs in the frying pan. Scramble the eggs by stirring them. Scramble the eggs and add the fish. Add an additional 2 minutes to the cooking. Serve.

Nutrition Calories: 205 Kcal, Proteins: 18.4g, Fat: 0.5g, Carbohydrates: 2.3g

3.9 Spinach and Potatoes with Smoked Salmon

Setup Time: 10 Minutes **Cooked in:** 0 Minutes **How many people:** 1 Person

Recipe Components:

- 2 russet potatoes (peeled and diced)
- 4 eggs
- 1/2 onion (sliced)
- 2 cups baby spinach (fresh)
- 8 ozs smoked salmon (sliced)
- 1/2 cup mushrooms (sliced)
- 2 tbsp olive oil
- 1 garlic clove (minced)
- 2 tbsp ghee
- 1/2 tsp garlic powder
- 1/2 tsp onion powder
- 1/4 tsp paprika
- Black pepper
- Sea salt

Preparation Steps: The oven has to be preheated to 425 degrees. Use parchment paper to line a baking dish. Put the potatoes in a single layer on the baking pan. Sprinkle paprika, olive oil, onion powder, and garlic powder over the potatoes. Put pepper on it. Russet potatoes need thirty minutes in the oven. At the halfway point, give the potatoes a flip. Heat water in a pot on high. Bring water to a boil and put the eggs in it. Remove heat. Leave eggs in hot water for 7 minutes. Take the eggs out of the cooker. The eggs should be rinsed under running water. Prepare the eggs by removing the shells. Put the ghee in a saucepan and melt it over a hob set that is somewhere in the middle. Warm the oil in a frying pan and then quickly sauté the garlic and onion in it for a few seconds. Put the mushrooms in the interior. You should season it with salt and pepper. Include an additional five minutes in the cooking section. Prepare the spinach and add it. Let them cook for 2 minutes or till they are crumpled. Cut the brown potatoes into quarters and serve them evenly. Pile smoked salmon on top of the eggs and spinach combination, and serve. Serve.

Nutrition Calories: 205 Kcal, Proteins: 6g, Fat: 2.1g, Carbohydrates: 2.3g

3.10 Eggs in a Mushroom and Bacon

Setup Time: 10 Minutes **Cooked in:** 0 Minutes **How many people:** 4 Persons

Recipe Components:

- 4 Portobello mushroom caps
- 4 pasture-raised eggs (large)
- 2 strips thick-cut and pasture-raised bacon (cooked and chopped)
- 1 cup arugula
- 1 medium tomato (chopped)
- Pepper
- Salt

Preparation Steps: Adjust the temperature in the oven to 350 degrees Fahrenheit. Therefore, get a baking sheet prepared. Place a piece of parchment paper inside of it. To get the mushroom heads off of the mushrooms, you can use a spoon. You should eliminate the gills. Spread the mushroom caps out in a single layer on the baking sheet that has been prepared.

Put some arugula and diced tomatoes in each mushroom cap and serve. Put an egg over mushroom stems very carefully. Put the mushrooms in the center of the oven and bake for 20 minutes. Put some bacon, salt, and pepper on top of each mushroom. Serve.

Nutrition Calories: 124 Kcal, Proteins: 8g, Fat: 8.4g, Carbohydrates: 4.3g

3.11 Bacon Avocado Burger

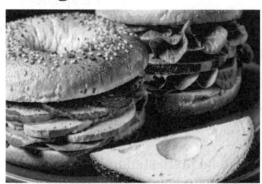

Setup Time: 10 Minutes **Cooked in:** 0 Minutes **How many people:** 1 Person

Recipe Components:

- 1 ripe avocado
- 2 bacon rashers
- 1 red onion (sliced)
- 1 lettuce leaf
- 1 egg
- Sea salt
- 1 tomato (sliced)
- Sesame seeds (for garnishing)
- 1 tbsp. Paleo mayonnaise

Preparation Steps: Carefully place the bacon in the pan. To preheat the stove, set the temperature to medium. Brown the bacon. Whenever the bacon rashers flare, flip them with a fork. Keep frying until they reach the desired crispiness. Don't eat any more of that deliciously crispy bacon right now. Break the egg into the same pan you used to cook the bacon. Make a fried egg in bacon grease. It is ideal for the egg white to be firm but the yolk to be soft. Put the finished egg to one side. You should halve the avocado lengthwise. Dig that hole out! Remove the meat by spooning it out of the skin. Spread the mayonnaise into the empty space left by the avocado. Spread the avocado on a plate, and then layer on the bacon, egg, tomato, and onion. Sprinkle some salt over it. Complete the layer by slicing the remaining avocado in half and spreading it on top. Sprinkle some sesame seeds on top. Serve.

Nutrition Calories: 440 Kcal, Proteins: 37g, Fat: 49g, Carbohydrates: 51g

3.12 Spinach Fry Up & Tomato Mushroom
Setup Time: 10 Minutes **Cooked in:** 5 Minutes **How many people:** 2 Persons

Recipe Components:

- 3 large handfuls of English spinach leaves (torn)
- 6 button mushrooms (sliced)
- A handful of cherry tomatoes (sliced in halves)
- 1 garlic clove (finely diced)
- Drizzle of lemon juice

- 1/2 red onion (sliced)
- 2 tbsp olive oil
- 1/2 tsp lemon zest (grated)
- 1 tsp ghee
- 1/2 tsp sea salt
- Pinch of black pepper (ground)
- Pinch of nutmeg

Preparation Steps: Put the olive oil and ghee in a pan and heat them over medium heat. The mushrooms and onions should be cooked in a sautéing pan until tender. Tomatoes, lemon, and garlic rind should be combined and stirred together. Add some salt, pepper, and nutmeg for flavor. Add an additional 2 minutes to the cooking. Make the minced tomato sauce by mashing tomatoes with a spatula. Add the spinach leaves and mix. Wilt them in the cooking process. Put some lime juice on it. Serve.

Nutrition Calories: 61.5 Kcal, Proteins: 3.3g, Fat: 2.5g, Carbohydrates: 6.6g

3.13 Chocolate Milkshake
Setup Time: 12 Minutes **Cooked in:** 5 Minutes **How many people:** 2 Persons

Recipe Components:

- 4 ice cubes
- 2 large organic bananas (frozen)
- 1/2 tsp vanilla extract
- 1 cup coconut milk
- 2 tbsp cashew butter
- 1 tbsp. cacao powder (raw)

Preparation Steps: Process the coconut cream and bananas in a blender until the mixture is completely smooth. Double or triple pulse. Stir in the cocoa powder, nut butter, and flavoring. Repeat the process two or three times. Fill it up with ice. Put everything in a blender and whir it up until it's completely combined. The consistency of the milkshake may be adjusted to taste by adding additional ice cubes or coconut milk. Fill a glass with it. Serve.

Nutrition Calories: 371 Kcal, Proteins: 8.2g, Fat: 17g, Carbohydrates: 51g

3.14 Almond Sweet Cherry Chia Pudding
Setup Time: 15 Minutes **Cooked in:** 0 Minutes **How many people:** 2 Persons

Recipe Components:

- 2 cups whole sweet cherries (pitted)
- 3/4 cup chia seeds
- 1/2 cup hemp seeds
- 1/4 cup maple syrup
- 13.5 oz can of coconut milk
- 1 tsp vanilla extract
- 1 tsp almond extract
- 1/8 tsp sea salt

Topping:

- four servings of cherry

Preparation Steps: The cherries, vanilla extract, coconut milk, almond extract, salt, and maple syrup should be blended together. They should be blended until they are completely smooth. Add the chia seeds and hemp seeds. Put everything in the blender and mix on a low speed to combine. Divide it across 4 glasses. Allow the pudding to chill in the refrigerator for a minimum of an hour. Cherry, each pudding to finish it off. Serve.

Nutrition Calories: 242 Kcal, Proteins: 7g, Fat: 11g, Carbohydrates: 33g

3.15 Shakshuka

Setup Time: 10 Minutes **Cooked in:** 12 Minutes **How many people:** 6 Persons

Recipe Components:

- 6 eggs (large)
- 4 cups tomatoes (diced)
- 1/2 onion (chopped)
- Sea salt
- 1 clove of garlic (minced)
- 1 red bell pepper (chopped and seeded)
- 2 tbsp tomato paste
- 1/2 tbsp. fresh parsley (finely chopped)
- 1 tbsp. cooking fat
- 1 tsp paprika
- Pinch of cayenne pepper
- 1 tsp chili powder
- Black pepper

Preparation Steps: Put the lard that will be used for frying in a pan and heat it over a medium fuel. The onions should be sautéed for two minutes. The garlic has to be added at this point. It is best to sauté the onions until they are completely tender. Add the red bell pepper and combine everything thoroughly. Hold off on serving the chills until they have reached the desired tenderness. Tomatoes, chili powder, paprika, cayenne pepper, and tomato paste should be stirred in. Add salt and pepper to taste. Temper the heat a little. The ingredients should be heated for several minutes at a low simmer. The eggs should be broken over the mixture while it is still boiling. Spread the eggs out equally. Keep the skillet covered. Maintain the heat until the eggs have reached the desired doneness. Sprinkle some chopped parsley on top.

Nutrition Calories: 298 Kcal, Proteins: 17g, Fat: 19g, Carbohydrates: 16g

3.16 Anti-Inflammatory Salad

Setup Time: 12 Minutes **Cooked in:** 0 Minutes **How many people:** 4 Persons

Recipe Components:

Dressing:

- 1 clove of garlic (grated)
- 1/3 cup extra virgin olive oil
- 2 tbsp apple cider vinegar
- 1 tbsp. lemon juice
- 1 tsp turmeric
- 1 tsp fresh ginger (grated)
- 1/2 tsp sea salt
- 1/4 tsp black pepper (freshly ground)

Salad:

- 16 ozs beets (cooked, peeled, and chopped)
- 2 12-ounce bags of Trader Joe's Sweet Kale Salad Mix
- 1 1/2 cup blueberries (fresh)

Preparation Steps: Put the dressing components in a blender and mix until smooth. The salad components should be split between six bowls. Dress with a drizzle. Serve.

Nutrition Calories: 20 Kcal, Proteins: 17g, Fat: 19g, Carbohydrates: 16g

3.17 Amaranth Porridge with Pears

Setup Time: 12 Minutes **Cooked in:** 5 Minutes **How many people:** 4 Persons

Recipe Components:

Pears:

- 1 tsp maple syrup
- 1 pear (large and diced)
- 1/2 tsp cinnamon (ground)
- 1/4 tsp ginger (ground)
- 1/8 tsp nutmeg (ground)
- 1/8 tsp clove (ground)

Porridge:

- 1/2 cup amaranth (uncooked, drained, and rinsed)
- 1/2 cup water
- 1 cup 2% milk
- 1/4 tsp salt

Topping:

- 1 cup 0% Greek yogurt (plain)
- 2 tbsp pecan pieces
- 1 tsp maple syrup (pure)

Preparation Steps: Raise the temperature in the oven to 400 degrees Fahrenheit. Prepare a baking pan by laying parchment paper on it. Prepare the porridge by placing all of the ingredients in a pot and cooking them over medium heat. When the water boiling, turn down the fuel. Allow the porridge to cook for a quarter of an hour. Putting aside. The pecan bits should be spread out on the prepared baking sheet. Spread maple syrup all over them. On the same baking sheet coated with pecan bits, place the diced pears. Pour some maple syrup over the pears. Bake them in the microwave for fifteen minutes. Stir the fruits into the cereal. Keep some pears for sprinkling. Two cups of porridge, please. Put some yogurt in each of the dishes. Porridge should be served in bowls. Add the remaining pears and pecans to the top of each serving of porridge. Serve.

Nutrition Calories: 500 Kcal, Proteins: 78g, Fat: 1.5g, Carbohydrates: 8g

3.18 Sweet Potato Breakfast Bowl

Setup Time: 15 Minutes **Cooked in:** 5 Minutes **How many people:** 3 Persons

Recipe Components:

- 1 small banana (sliced)
- 1 small sweet potato (pre-baked)
- 1/4 cup raspberries
- 1 serving protein powder
- 1/4 cup blueberries

Toppings:

- Favorite nuts
- Chia seeds
- Cacao nibs
- Hemp hearts

Preparation Steps: Purée the sweet potato in a bowl. Add the protein powder and mix well. Mix. Arrange the bananas, raspberries, and blueberries on top. Sprinkle on the condiments after.

Nutrition Calories: 210 Kcal, Proteins: 3.8g, Fat: 1.3g, Carbohydrates: 48g

3.19 Apple Turkey Hash

Setup Time: 20 Minutes **Cooked in:** 0 Minutes **How many people:** 4 Persons

Recipe Components:

Hash:

- 2 cups spinach
- 2 cups frozen butternut squash (cubed)
- 1/2 cup carrots (shredded)
- 1 large apple (peeled, cored, and chopped)
- 1 onion
- 1 large zucchini
- 1 tsp cinnamon
- 1 tbsp. coconut oil
- 1/2 tsp thyme (dried)
- 1/2 tsp garlic powder
- 1/2 tsp turmeric
- 3/4 tsp powdered ginger
- Sea salt

Meat:

- 1/2 tsp thyme (dried)
- 1 pound ground turkey
- 1 tbsp. coconut oil
- 1/2 tsp cinnamon
- Sea salt

Preparation Steps: Take the coconut oil in a saucepan and warm it up over a heat setting of medium. When the turkey is done cooking, add it to the pan with the other ingredients and mix it in. To enhance the flavour, sprinkle on additional salt, pepper, cinnamon, and thyme. Place the coconut oil in the same pan and heat it over a temperature that is considered to be moderate. Sautéing the onions will make them more refined. Mix in the apples, butternut squash, carrots, and zucchini. Make sure they're cooked all the way through so they're nice and tender. Blend in the spinach. If you want it wilted, cook it longer. Add the minced turkey and mix it with the other ingredients. Serve.

Nutrition Calories: 325 Kcal, Proteins: 28g, Fat: 19g, Carbohydrates: 20g

3.20 Oats with Almonds and Blueberries

Setup Time: 15 Minutes **Cooked in:** 0 Minutes **How many people:** 4 Persons

Recipe Components:

Oats:

- 3/4 cup old-fashioned oats
- 3/4 cup almond milk
- 1 tbsp. maple syrup

Toppings:

- 1/4 cup blueberries
- 1/3 cup yogurt
- 3 tbsp almonds (sliced)

Preparation Steps: Put the oats in a canning jar that holds one pint of liquid. In a bowl, thoroughly mix together the almond milk and the maple syrup. Combine the honey and milk before adding it to the oats. Make sure the lid is secure in the jar.

Put it in the fridge for at least eight hours, ideally overnight, and save it. Fill it with condiments. Serve.

Nutrition Calories: 230 Kcal, Proteins: 8g, Fat: 5g, Carbohydrates: 40g

3.21 Chia Energy Bars with Chocolate
Setup Time: 12 Minutes **Cooked in:** 0 Minutes **How many people:** 4 Persons

Recipe Components:

- 1 cup walnut pieces (raw)
- 1 1/2 cups pitted dates (packed)
- 1/3 cup cacao powder (raw)
- 1/2 cup whole chia seeds
- 1/2 cup coconut shavings
- 1 tsp pure vanilla extract
- 1/2 cup dark chocolate (chopped)
- 1/4 tsp sea salt (unrefined)
- 1/2 cup oats

Preparation Steps: Place the dates into the food processor. Prepare a thick paste by processing. Place it in a basin for mixing. Drop the walnuts in there. Ensure an in-depth blending. Add the last of the ingredients. Knead it until it creates a ball of dough. Obtain a square dish for baking. Prepare the dish by lining it with baking parchment. Put the mixture on the baking sheet that has been prepared. Distribute the dough in an even layer, and after that, press it down firmly into the dish. Freeze for at least a few hours and up to a full day. Cube into 14 pieces. Serve.

Nutrition Calories: 234 Kcal, Proteins: 4.5g, Fat: 12g, Carbohydrates: 28g

3.22 Baked Rice Porridge with Maple and Fruit
Setup Time: 15 Minutes **Cooked in:** 0 Minutes **How many people:** 5 Persons

Recipe Components:

- 2 tbsp pure maple syrup
- 1/2 cup brown rice
- 1/2 tsp pure vanilla extract
- Pinch of cinnamon
- Sliced fruits (berries, plums, pears, or cherries)
- Pinch of salt

Preparation Steps: Raise the temperature in the oven to 400 degrees Fahrenheit. In a pot, over moderate heat, brown rice and a glass of water should be cooked together until the rice is done. Get the water boiling. Blend with some vanilla bean paste and cinnamon. Cover. Turn down the fuel. Allow the rice to boil until it is done. Toss the rice every once in a while. Have two bowls that can go from fridge to oven ready. Assign each bowl the same amount of rice. Sprinkle some maple syrup and sliced fruits over the rice. Put some salt on it. Put in the oven and set the timer for 15 minutes. Serve.

Nutrition Calories: 228 Kcal, Proteins: 3.5g, Fat: 1.5g, Carbohydrates: 50g

3.23 Banana Chia Pudding

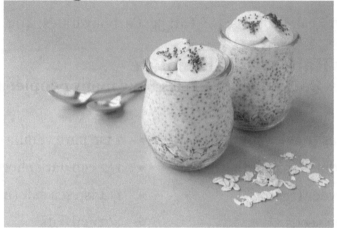

Setup Time: 20 Minutes **Cooked in:** 0 Minutes **How many people:** 5 Persons

Recipe Components:

- 1/2 cup chia seeds
- 2 cups almond milk (unsweetened)
- 1 large banana (very ripe)

- 1/2 tsp pure vanilla extract
- 2 tbsp. maple syrup
- 1 tbsp. cacao powder

Mix-ins:

- 2 tbsp chocolate chips
- 2 tbsp cacao nibs

- 1 large banana (sliced)

Preparation Steps: Place the mashed banana and chia seeds in a large bowl and mix them together until they are well combined. Combine the components by thoroughly mashing them together. Blend the milk and vanilla extract together before adding it to the pan. Be sure to thoroughly combine all of the ingredients. Get two sealed containers ready. To divide the chia seeds in half, divide the mixture between two containers. Cover. The remaining portion of the hemp seeds combination should be combined with maple syrup and cacao powder. Check that everything is well mixed together. Move the substance over to the second container. Avoid the sun. These containers need to be stored in the refrigerator for a minimum of a few hours and preferably for the entire night. Divide the chia pudding and the toppings into 3 glasses and layer. Serve.

Nutrition Calories: 260 Kcal, Proteins: 6g, Fat: 5g, Carbohydrates: 60g

3.24 Baked Eggs with Herbs
Setup Time: 15 Minutes **Cooked in:** 10 Minutes **How many people:** 5 Persons

Recipe Components:

- A tbsp. of milk
- A sprinkling of dried herbs like thyme, oregano, parsley, garlic powder, and dill
- A tsp of melted butter,
- Two eggs

Preparation Steps: Turn the oven's broiler on to a low level and preheat it. Put the butter and milk in a medium baking dish. Combo together successfully. Spread the butter-milk combo all over the baking dish. Separate the eggs and place them in the dish. Top with a sprinkling of herbs and garlic. Put it in the oven for a couple of minutes so the eggs can bake.

Nutrition Calories: 341 Kcal, Proteins: 20g, Fat: 27g, Carbohydrates: 3g

3.25 Banana Bread Pecan Overnight Oats
Setup Time: 20 Minutes **Cooked in:** 0 Minutes **How many people:** 5 Persons

Recipe Components:

- 1 cup old-fashioned rolled oats
- 1 1/2 cups milk
- 1/4 cup Greek yogurt (plain)
- 2 tbsp honey
- 2 bananas (very ripe, mashed)

- 2 tbsp coconut flakes
- 1/4 tsp sea salt (flaked)
- 1 tbsp. chia seeds
- 2 tsps vanilla extract

Topping:

- Banana slices
- Roasted pecans
- Honey

- Pomegranate seeds
- Fig halves

Preparation Steps: To make, in a large mixing bowl, combine the oats, coconut flakes, bananas, milk, yogurt, honey, chia seeds, vanilla extract, and sea salt essence. Blend together well. Place the oat mixture into two bowls and divide it in half. Cover. The recommended minimum time in the fridge is 6 hours but overnight is best. Toss the ingredients together and stir. Add the toppings to each plate of oats and serve. Serve.

Nutrition Calories: 370 Kcal, Proteins: 16g, Fat: 8g, Carbohydrates: 58g

3.26 Cinnamon Granola with Fruits
Setup Time: 15 Minutes **Cooked in:** 0 Minutes **How many people:** 5 Persons

Recipe Components:

- 1/4 cup walnuts (chopped)
- 2 cups old-fashioned rolled oats
- 1/4 cup shredded coconut (unsweetened)
- 1/4 cup dried apricots (chopped)
- 1/4 cup honey
- 1/4 cup raisins

- 4 tbsp unsalted butter (melted)
- 1/4 tsp ground cloves
- 1/4 cup dried cranberries
- 2 tbsp pumpkin seeds
- 1/4 tsp ground nutmeg
- 1/2 tsp ground cinnamon

Preparation Steps: Raise the temperature inside the oven to three hundred degrees Fahrenheit. Putting parchment paper on a baking sheet is the first step in getting it ready for use. In a large mixing bowl, combine the oats, pumpkin seeds, spices, coconuts, walnuts, and salt all at the same time. It is not worth your time to deal with it at this time.

Throw the honey and butter into a separate bowl. Combo together successfully. After the liquid has been added to the oats, mix well. Place the oat mixture on the baking sheet that has been prepared. The distribution has to be even throughout. Bake for 20 to 25 minutes once it's been put in the oven. Let it cool down a little. Prepare the granola by breaking it up. Combine the granola pieces and dried fruit. Put away in a container with a tight lid.

Nutrition Calories: 120 Kcal, Proteins: 2g, Fat: 4.5g, Carbohydrates: 18g

3.27 Yogurt Parfait with Chia Seeds and Raspberries
Setup Time: 20 Minutes **Cooked in:** 0 Minutes **How many people:** 5 Persons

Recipe Components:

- 16 ozs yogurt (plain, divided into 4 portions)
- 1/2 cup raspberries (fresh)
- 2 tbsp chia seeds
- 1 tsp maple syrup
- Pinch of cinnamon

Topping:

- Nectarines (sliced)
- Strawberries (sliced)
- Blackberries (sliced)

Preparation Steps: Put the raspberries in a big bowl or other container. Mix them together and mash them up until they have the consistency of jam. Mix with some cinnamon and honey with some chia seeds. Put everything in a blender and blitz it until it's a uniform consistency. Divide into halves and set aside. Put two in the glass. Spread some yogurt on the bottom of each cup. The raspberry filling comes next. The last layer consists of any leftover yogurt. Incorporate the condiments. Serve.

Nutrition Calories: 252 Kcal, Proteins: 13g, Fat: 12g, Carbohydrates: 25g

3.28 Avocado Toast with Egg
Setup Time: 15 Minutes **Cooked in:** 10 Minutes **How many people:** 4 Persons

Recipe Components:

- 1 slice of gluten-free bread (toasted)
- 1 1/2 tsp ghee
- 1 egg (scrambled)
- Red pepper flakes
- 1/2 avocado (sliced)
- A handful of spinach leaves

Preparation Steps: Apply some ghee to the hot toast. Layer the toast with avocado slices. Spinach leaves are a great garnish. The scrambled egg should be served on top. Add some crushed red pepper for heat. Serve.

Nutrition Calories: 260 Kcal, Proteins: 12g, Fat: 16g, Carbohydrates: 20g

3.29 Winter Morning Breakfast Bowl
Setup Time: 15 Minutes **Cooked in:** 0 Minutes **How many people:** 4 Persons

Recipe Components:

- 1 cup of quinoa
- 2 1/2 cups coconut water

- 2 whole cloves
- 1-star anise pod

- 1 cinnamon stick

Fresh Fruits:

- Blackberries
- Apples
- Cranberries

- Persimmons
- Pears

Preparation Steps: In a saucepan, combine the coconut water, quinoa, and spices, and bring the mixture to a simmer over medium heat. Keep stirring them occasionally until they reach a full boil. Put the lid on it. Turn down the stove. The recommended cooked time is 25 minutes. Split the quinoa in half and place it in separate dishes. Do not use entire spices. Put some fruit on top of each dish. Serve.

Nutrition Calories: 257 Kcal, Proteins: 12g, Fat: 8g, Carbohydrates: 40g

3.30 Broccoli and Quinoa Breakfast Patties
Setup Time: 5 Minutes **Cooked in:** 6 Minutes **How many people:** 3 Persons

Recipe Components:

- 1/2 cup shredded broccoli florets
- 1 cup cooked quinoa, cooked
- 1/2 cup shredded carrots
- 2 tsp parsley
- 2 cloves of garlic, minced
- 1 1/2 tsp onion powder

- 1/3 tsp salt
- 1 1/2 tsp garlic powder
- 1/4 tsp black pepper
- 2 tbsp. coconut oil
- 1/2 cup bread crumbs, gluten-free
- 2 flax eggs

Preparation Steps: Please take all of the ingredients, save the oil, into a large bowl, and whisk them together until they are entirely smooth. In order to do the patties, heat the oil in a pan over moderate heat. Once the oil has reached the desired temperature, add the patties to the skillet. Cook the patties for about three minutes on each side, and then remove them from the fire. Prepare vegan sour creams to accompany the burgers.

Nutrition Calories: 190 Kcal, Proteins: 9g, Fat: 5g, Carbohydrates: 23g

3.31 Scrambled Tofu Breakfast Tacos
Setup Time: 5 Minutes **Cooked in:** 10 Minutes **How many people:** 4 Persons

Recipe Components:

- 1/2 cup grape tomatoes, quartered
- 12 ozs tofu, pressed, drained
- 1 medium red pepper, diced
- 1 clove of garlic, minced
- 8 corn tortillas
- 1 medium avocado, sliced

- 1/4 tsp ground turmeric
- 1 tsp olive oil
- 1/4 tsp salt
- 1/4 tsp ground black pepper
- 1/4 tsp cumin

Preparation Steps: When the oil has reached the desired temperature, add the garlic and pepper to the pan and continue to cook for another two minutes. Heat the oil in a skillet over a moderate burner. Add some crumbled tofu, then season it with salt, black pepper, and the rest of the ingredients. Cook it for five minutes while turning it regularly and flavoring it with salt and pepper. When everything is finished, split the tofu between the tortillas and top each one with some tomato and avocado.

Nutrition Calories: 240 Kcal, Proteins: 12g, Fat: 8g, Carbohydrates: 26g

3.32 Potato Skillet Breakfast
Setup Time: 5 Minutes **Cooked in:** 15 Minutes **How many people:** 5 Persons

Recipe Components:

- 1 1/4 pounds potatoes, diced
- 1 ½ cup cooked black beans
- 12 ozs spinach
- 2 small avocados, sliced, for topping
- 1 1/4 pounds red potatoes, diced
- 1 medium green bell pepper, diced
- 1 large white onion, diced
- 1 jalapeno, minced
- 1 medium red bell pepper, diced
- 1/2 tsp red chili powder
- 3 cloves of garlic, minced
- 1/4 tsp salt
- 1 tbsp. canola oil
- 1 tsp cumin

Preparation Steps: Turn on the oven and adjust the temperature to 425 degrees Fahrenheit; the dish will be ready in a short while if it has been warmed. The second step is to put the oil in a pan and heat it over medium-low heat. After the oil has been heated, add the potatoes and fry them for two minutes while tossing them often. After that, season the potatoes with salt, chilli powder, and cumin. Put the pan in the microwave and bake the potatoes for twenty minutes, giving them a stir once halfway through the cooking process, until they are cooked through. After the first 15 minutes, add the remaining bell peppers, onion, garlic, and jalapeno to the roasting pan and continue to cook, turning the pan over once halfway through. Put the pan on the stove over moderate heat, and cook the potatoes for five to ten minutes, tossing them regularly until they are soft. After adding the beans and spinach, continue to boil for another three minutes, stirring the mixture regularly until the basil leaves have wilted. When everything is done, garnish the skillet with chopped cilantro and serve it with avocado.

Nutrition Calories: 199 Kcal, Proteins: 4g, Fat: 7g, Carbohydrates: 32g

3.33 Peanut Butter and Banana Bread Granola
Setup Time: 10 Minutes **Cooked in:** 32 Minutes **How many people:** 6 Persons

Recipe Components:

- 1/2 cup mashed banana
- 1/2 cup Quinoa
- 3 cup rolled oats, old-fashioned
- 1 cup peanuts, salted
- 1 cup banana chips, crushed
- 1 tsp. salt
- 1/4 cup brown sugar
- 1 tsp. cinnamon
- 1/4 cup honey
- 1/3 cup peanut butter
- 2 tsps. vanilla extract, unsweetened
- 6 tbsp. unsalted butter

Preparation Steps: Turn on the microwave and prepare it for 325 degrees Fahrenheit. Prepare two lined baking trays ahead of time by lining them with parchment paper and setting them away. Stir together the oats, banana chips, quinoa, cinnamon, sugar, and salt in a bowl. Place the butter and honey in a small saucepan and cook them over a low temperature, stirring often, for approximately four minutes or until the honey has melted completely. After that, remove the pan from the heat and stir in the bananas and vanilla extract until everything is thoroughly blended. At last, include this component into the grain mixture while continuing to stir. When the granola has reached the desired colour, which should be golden brown, remove it from the oven and divide the mixture evenly between two baking pans. Cool the granola completely on the baking sheets set over wire racks before breaking it up and serving. As soon as possible, serve.

Nutrition Calories: 655 Kcal, Proteins: 18g, Fat: 36g, Carbohydrates: 70g

3.34 Chocolate Chip, Strawberry and Oat Waffles
Setup Time: 10 Minutes **Cooked in:** 25 Minutes **How many people:** 6 Persons

Recipe Components:

- 6 tbsp chocolate chips, semi-sweet
- 1/4 tsp salt
- ½ cup chopped strawberries
- 2 tsps baking powder

Wet Recipe Components:

1. 1/3 cup mashed bananas
2. Powdered sugar as needed for topping

Dry Recipe Components:

- 1/4 cup oats
- 2 tbsp. maple syrup
- 2 tbsp. coconut oil
- 1/2 tsp vanilla extract, unsweetened
- 1 1/2 tbsp. ground flaxseeds
- 1 1/2 cup whole wheat pastry flour
- 2 1/2 tbsp. cocoa powder
- 1/4 cup applesauce, unsweetened
- 1 3/4 cup almond milk, unsweetened

Preparation Steps: Place the dry ingredients in a bowl of a suitable size and whisk them together to combine. Place the liquid ingredients in a basin of a suitable size and stir them thoroughly until they are combined. After adding the dry ingredients, whisk them in four consecutive batches until the mixture is completely smooth. In the meanwhile, turn on the griddle and let it heat up to a high temperature while you let the batter sit out at ambient temperature for Five minutes. Then, spoon in a sixth of the mixture and bake until the pancake is firm and golden. Keep making waffles in a similar fashion until all the batter is gone, then sprinkle the finished waffles with sugar and top with cocoa powder and fruit.

Nutrition Calories: 261 Kcal, Proteins: 6g, Fat: 10g, Carbohydrates: 41g

3.35 Chickpea Flour Omelet
Setup Time: 5 Minutes **Cooked in:** 12 Minutes **How many people:** 1 Person

Recipe Components:

- Approximately one-half of a tsp of chopped chives
- 1/4 cup of chickpea flour

- 1/2 cup of chopped spinach
- 1/4 tsp. of garlic powder
- Exactly a Cup and a Tbsp. of Water
- A pinch of turmeric
- Black pepper, ground, 1/8 tsp
- 1/2 tsp of yeast extract
- The equivalent of half a tsp of baking powder
- 1/2 tsp. egg substitute for vegans

Preparation Steps: Everything else, including the spinach, should be put in a bowl and whisked together to combine. Put to the side for the next 5 minutes. After that, warm some oil in a skillet by placing it over a low heat source. After the pan has reached the desired temperature, add the ingredients and allow them to simmer for three minutes or until the edges become dry. After that, spread spinach over one half of the omelette, fold the other half over it, and continue cooking for another two minutes. The omelet should be slid onto a platter and served with ketchup.

Nutrition Calories: 151 Kcal, Proteins: 10g, Fat: 2g, Carbohydrates: 24g

CHAPTER 4: Anti-Inflammatory Lunch Recipes

4.1 Buddha Bowl with Avocado, Wild Rice, Kale, and Orange
Setup Time: 15 Minutes **Cooked in:** 12 Minutes **How many people:** 4 Persons

Recipe Components:

Rice:

- 1 cup wild rice
- 3 cups vegetable broth
- 1 garlic clove (minced)
- 2 tbsp extra-virgin olive oil
- 2 tbsp rice vinegar
- 1 tbsp. fresh mint (chopped)
- Salt
- Freshly ground black pepper

Toppings:

- 1/4 cup pumpkin seeds
- 1/4 cup pomegranate seeds
- 1 bunch kale (roughly chopped)
- Salt
- 1 orange (segmented)
- 2 eggs (hard-boiled)
- 1/2 avocado (sliced)
- 2 tbsp olive oil
- 1 tbsp. rice vinegar
- Freshly ground black pepper

Preparation Steps: Rice: Take the rice and garlic, stock in a pot, and cook on low heat for ten minutes. Stir the ingredients together to combine. Bring it to a boil. Reduce the heat, please. Rice needs at least fifteen minutes on the hob at a low simmer to get fully cooked and absorb all of the liquid. The rice will be more manageable to eat if you wait 10 minutes to serve it. Toss with some mint, olive oil, vinegar, salt, and pepper. Toss with the rice until evenly combined. **Toppings:** Mix the kale, olive oil, and vinegar together in a big basin. Give it a spin to combine the ingredients. Separate the rice into two serving bowls. Each serving of rice should be topped with the kale mixture. Distribute the remaining condiments fairly between the two serving bowls. Spice things up with some salt and pepper. Serve.

Nutrition Calories: 1059 Kcal, Proteins: 65g, Fat: 38g, Carbohydrates: 108g

4.2 Avocado Chickpea Salad Sandwich
Setup Time: 12 Minutes **Cooked in:** 15 Minutes **How many people:** 6 Persons

Recipe Components:

- 1 15-ounce-can chickpea (drained and rinsed)
- 1 large avocado (ripe)
- Freshly ground pepper
- 2 tsps lime juice
- 1/4 cup cranberries (dried)
- 4 slices of whole grain bread
- Salt

Toppings:

- Arugula
- Red onion
- Spinach

Preparation Steps: Put the chickpeas in a big basin and stir them around. Use a fork to mix them up. Prepare the avocado by placing it inside. Keep crushing it until it's mostly fine with some lumpy bits. Cranberries and fresh lemon juice should be added. Add some salt and pepper for flavor. Combine in a harmonious manner. The bread should be toasted. The chickpea mixture should be divided in half. Spread one serving onto a piece of toast. Apply your preferred toppings on the top. Add another piece of bread to finish the sandwich. Serve.

Nutrition Calories: 340 Kcal, Proteins: 15g, Fat: 12g, Carbohydrates: 46g

4.3 Spiced Lentil Soup

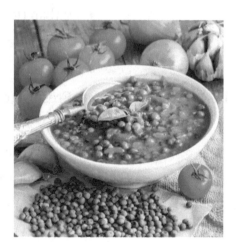

Setup Time: 20 Minutes **Cooked in:** 20 Minutes **How many people:** 4 Persons

Recipe Components:

- 3/4 cup red lentils (rinsed, uncooked, and drained)
- 3 1/2 cups vegetable broth (low-sodium)
- 1 1/2 tbsp extra-virgin olive oil
- 1 large onion (diced)
- 2 garlic cloves (minced)
- Freshly ground black pepper
- Two 14-ounce-cans: one of coconut milk (full-fat) and another of diced tomatoes (with juice)

- 1 5-ounce-package baby spinach
- Ground spices: 2 tsps turmeric, 1 1/2 tsps cumin, 1/4 tsp cardamom, and 1/2 tsp cinnamon
- 2 tsps fresh lime juice
- Seasonings: 1/2 tsp fine sea salt and a dash of cayenne pepper

Preparation Steps: Put the oil into a pan and heat it over medium heat. To soften the onion, sauté it with garlic and salt. Cardamom, turmeric, cumin, and cinnamon should be added now. Combine ingredients by stirring. Continue cooking for one minute. Mix in the red lentils, broth, cayenne pepper, black pepper, coconut milk, and salt. Mix well by stirring. Let the liquid reach a rolling boil. Turn down the stove. Allow the ingredients to boil for twenty minutes. Take it away from the stove. Do not forget the spinach! Combine ingredients by stirring. Add some salt, pepper, and lime juice for seasoning. Serve.

Nutrition Calories: 331 Kcal, Proteins: 30g, Fat: 3.6g, Carbohydrates: 47.5g

4.4 Red Lentil Pasta with Tomato

Setup Time: 15 Minutes **Cooked in:** 10 Minutes **How many people:** 4 Persons

Recipe Components:

- 1/4 cup extra virgin olive oil
- 1/2 cup sun-dried tomatoes (oil-packed, drained, and chopped)
- 6 cloves garlic (minced)
- 2 large handfuls of kale
- 1 sweet onion (chopped)
- 1 can (28 ozs) fire roasted tomatoes
- 1 tbsp. oregano (dried)
- 1 box (8 ozs) of red lentil pasta
- 1 tbsp. basil (dried)
- 2 tsps turmeric (ground)
- 1 tbsp. apple cider vinegar
- Pepper
- Toasted pine nuts (for topping)
- Kosher salt

Preparation Steps: Heat the oil in a pan on a hob between low and medium heat. To get the onion to the appropriate softness, sauté it for about five minutes. After that, you'll want to combine ingredients like garlic, basil, oregano, turmeric, salt, and pepper. Don't stop cooking for another minute. Please include the juice with the roasted tomatoes. Break up the tomatoes by stirring them thoroughly. Sun-dried tomatoes and balsamic vinegar should be added to this. Simmer the liquid for 15 minutes, with the pot set over low heat. Toss the greens in and mix it up. 5 additional minutes of cooking are required. The red lentil spaghetti should be prepared as directed on the box. Divide the spaghetti into 6 bowls into equal amounts. Sprinkle some pine nuts and tomato sauce on top of each bowl. Serve.

Nutrition Calories: 270 Kcal, Proteins: 8.5g, Fat: 4.5g, Carbohydrates: 49g

4.5 Tuna Mediterranean Salad

Setup Time: 15 Minutes **Cooked in:** 05 Minutes **How many people:** 4 Persons

Recipe Components:

- Two cans: one 14.5-ounce-can chickpea (drained and rinsed) and 2 cans of Albacore Tuna (drained)
- 1 cup red peppers (roasted and chopped)
- 1/2 cup pepperoncini (diced)
- Chopped ingredients: 1/3 cup parsley (finely) and 1/4 cup feta cheese
- 1 cucumber (chopped)
- 1/2 red onion (diced)
- 2 tsps capers
- Pinch of fine sea salt
- Sundried tomatoes (chopped)
- Olives
- Pinch of black pepper

Dressing:

- 2 tbsp each: olive oil and red wine vinegar
- 1 tsp each: lemon juice, dried parsley, and dried oregano
- Pinches: black pepper and fine salt

Preparation Steps: Put everything for the salad into a large mixing basin. Throw everything for the dressing into a separate dish. Stir the whisk vigorously. Coat the salad with the dressing. Throw everything together in a bowl and toss. Serve with half of an avocado.

Nutrition Calories: 230 Kcal, Proteins: 28g, Fat: 10g, Carbohydrates: 40g

4.6 Chicken and Greek Salad Wrap
Setup Time: 15 Minutes **Cooked in:** 25 Minutes **How many people:** 2 Persons

Recipe Components:

- 1 tbsp. olive oil (divided)

- 2 chicken breasts (bone-in)

- 1/2 tsp each: dried oregano, lemon pepper, and garlic powder

Salad:

- 1/3 cup each: feta cheese and cherry tomatoes (sliced)

- 4 cups romaine (chopped)

- 1/4 cup red onion

- 1/2 cup cucumber slices (chopped)

- 2 tbsp each: kalamata olives and hummus

- 4 tbsp gluten-free wraps

- Seasonings: red wine vinegar, olive oil, 1/2 tsp dried oregano, and 1 fresh lemon wedge (juiced)

Preparation Steps: Salad: Mix the romaine, cucumbers, tomatoes, onions, oregano, cheese, and olives on a serving dish. Make a dressing for the salad using the juice of half a lemon, one turn of the canola oil, and two tsps of vinegar. Synergizing through tossing. **Chicken:** Starting the oven is the first step in baking at 375 degrees Fahrenheit. Get some foil ready for a baking pan. Make do with roughly a third of the recommended olive oil. The prepared baking sheet is where you have to put the chicken. We recommend seasoning it with salt, pepper, pepper flakes, garlic powder, oregano, and lemon pepper. Add the remaining olive oil by drizzling it over the ingredients. To bake, set oven temperature to 400 degrees and wait 40 minutes. The chicken should be completely chilled before being served. Doing easy manipulable pieces. **Wrap:** Smear each wrap with 2 tbsp of hummus. Add the salad and chicken pieces in layers. Wrap. Serve.

Nutrition Calories: 230 Kcal, Proteins: 39g, Fat: 28g, Carbohydrates: 22g

4.7 Cauliflower and Chickpea Coconut Curry
Setup Time: 15 Minutes **Cooked in:** 25 Minutes **How many people:** 2 Persons

Recipe Components:

- Two cans: 1 can (14 ozs) of coconut milk and 1 can (28 ozs) of cooked chickpeas

- 1 1/2 cups frozen peas

- Thinly sliced: 4 scallions, 1 red onion, and 1 red bell pepper

- 1 lime (halved)

- 1 small head cauliflower (bite-size florets)
- 3 tbsp red curry paste
- 1 tbsp each: extra-virgin olive oil and fresh ginger (minced)
- Minced: 3 garlic cloves and 1/4 cup fresh cilantro
- Seasonings: salt, freshly ground black pepper, 1 tsp ground coriander, and 2 tsps chili powder

Preparation Steps: Prepare a pan with oil and set it over medium heat. Bell peppers and onions need to be cooked for 5 minutes. Add some ginger and garlic to the meal. Keep stirring for a full minute. You may spice things up by adding some coriander, cabbage, curry paste, or chili powder. Hold on a second. Put in the coconut milk and heat it up. Stir. When the cauliflower is soft, remove it from the fire and discard the bay leaf. Lime juice should be added to the curry. Stir. Include the chickpeas and peas. Add some salt and pepper for flavor. Just let it a few minutes to boil. Sprinkle a spoonful of scallions and parsley over each serving. Serve.

Nutrition Calories: 442 Kcal, Proteins: 15g, Fat: 12g, Carbohydrates: 33g

4.8 Butternut Squash Carrot Soup
Setup Time: 20 Minutes **Cooked in:** 15 Minutes **How many people:** 4 Persons

Recipe Components:

- Chopped: 1 pound of carrots and 1 1/2 pounds of butternut squash (peeled)
- 4 cups vegetable stock
- 1 can coconut milk (full-fat)
- 1/2 cup shallots (sliced)
- 2 tbsp each: avocado oil and 1 tbsp. fresh ginger (grated)
- Seasonings: 1 tsp salt and freshly ground black pepper

Garnishing:

- Roasted chickpeas
- Coconut milk
- Cilantro

Preparation Steps: Turn the oven temperature up to 400 degrees F. Spread parchment paper on a baking pan. Scatter the carrots, butternut squash, and shallots on the prepared baking sheet. Add oil and drizzle. Add some salt. Give the veggies a little toss to coat. Put them in the oven for 30 minutes at 375 degrees. Give them a few minutes to calm off. Combine the roasted veggies, vegetable stock, coconut milk, ginger, salt, and pepper in a blender. A creamy consistency may be achieved by blending. Put some soup in each of the four bowls. Top each serving with chickpeas, coconut milk, and cilantro.

Nutrition Calories: 129 Kcal, Proteins: 6.5g, Fat: 2.7g, Carbohydrates: 23g

4.9 Kale Quinoa Shrimp Bowl
Setup Time: 25 Minutes **Cooked in:** 30 Minutes **How many people:** 4 Persons

Recipe Components:

Quinoa:

- 1 1/4 cups quinoa
- 2 cups chicken broth

- 2 tsps extra-virgin olive oil

Kale:

- 2 tbsp extra-virgin olive oil
- Salt

Shrimp and Toppings:

- Thinly sliced: 2 watermelon radishes and 2 avocados
- 1 pound shrimp (cleaned and deveined)
- 1 tbsp. extra-virgin olive oil
- 2 tbsp hot sauce

- Seasonings: Salt and freshly ground pepper

- 1 bunch lacinato kale (roughly torn)
- Freshly ground black pepper

- Ground spices: 3/4 tsp coriander, 1 tsp cumin
- Seasonings: Salt and a dash of freshly ground black pepper

Preparation Steps: Quinoa: In a saucepan, warm the olive oil over low to medium heat. The quinoa should be mixed together in a complete mixture. One minute of toasting. Combine with the fluid. The quinoa must be boiled for 15 minutes to ensure it is fully cooked. Season with salt and pepper to taste. **Kale:** Adjust the oven temperature up to 400 degrees F. Prepare a parchment paper-lined baking sheet. The kale and olive oil should be combined in a large basin. Improve the flavor with some salt and pepper. Simply toss into a mashup. Spread the kale in a single layer on a baking sheet and toss with the olive oil. You should cook your meal for 15 minutes if you want it to be particularly crispy. **Shrimp and Toppings:** Olive oil should be heated in a pan over moderate heat. Combine the shrimp, spicy sauce, salt, and pepper in a mixing bowl. Add the cumin and cilantro. Simply toss into a mashup. In a pan over medium heat, the shrimp combination is cooked for 5 minutes. Distribute the quinoa among four bowls. Crispy kale, avocado chunks, watermelon radishes, and shrimp all make delicious additions to the soup. To aid.

Nutrition Calories: 377 Kcal, Proteins: 37g, Fat: 7g, Carbohydrates: 436g

---

4.10 Egg Bowl and Veggies

Setup Time: 15 Minutes **Cooked in:** 05 Minutes **How many people:** 4 Persons

Recipe Components:

- Cut vegetables: 1 pound Brussels sprouts (halved) and 1 pound sweet potatoes (cubed)
- 4 eggs (prepared poached)

- Liquid seasonings: 1 1/2 tbsp olive oil and 3 tbsp apple cider vinegar
- 2 cups arugula
- 2 tbsp harissa

Preparation Steps: Start the oven and heat it to 450 degrees Fahrenheit. Line a baking sheet with parchment paper. Spread the sweet potatoes and Brussels sprouts out in a single layer on the baking pan. Add some olive oil and mix it up. Boost the taste with some salt and pepper, for 20 minutes at 400 degrees Fahrenheit, or until meat is tender. Whisk together the harissa, olive oil, and apple cider vinegar. Prepare four individual servings of roasted vegetables. Top each serving with arugula, harissa, and an egg dressing. Serve.

Nutrition Calories: 263 Kcal, Proteins: 16g, Fat: 20g, Carbohydrates: 4.6g

4.11 Turkey Taco Bowls

Setup Time: 20 Minutes **Cooked in:** 15 Minutes **How many people:** 2 Persons

Recipe Components:

Turkey:

- 2/3 cup water
- 3/4 pound ground turkey (lean)
- 2 tbsp taco seasoning

Salsa:

- Chopped ingredients: 1/4 cup red onion, 1-pint cherry tomatoes (cut in half), and 1 jalapeno
- 1/2 lime for juicing
- 1/8 tsp salt

Rice:

- 3/4 cup brown rice (uncooked)
- 1/8 tsp salt
- 1 lime (zested)

Topping:

- 1 can (12 ozs) of corn kernels (drained)
- 1/2 cup mozzarella (shredded)

Preparation Steps: Follow the package directions for cooking the brown rice. It's as simple as seasoning the boiling water with salt and lime zest. Put the hot rice in a separate bowl to cool down. Put the turkey into a skillet and cook it over medium heat. Leave the turkey in the oven for 10 minutes or until it's no pinker inside. Add the water and taco seasoning to the pot. Combine ingredients by stirring. Keep the pot on low heat for two min to smooth the sauce. The turkey has to be chilled in cold water. In a large bowl, combine all of the salsa's components. Combine well and mix. Put some rice on each of the four plates. Turkey and salsa may be used as toppings for the rice bowls. Scatter the corn kernels and mozzarella over the top. Serve.

Nutrition Calories: 580 Kcal, Proteins: 26g, Fat: 25g, Carbohydrates: 62g

---

4.12 Bulgur Kale Pesto Salad

Setup Time: 10 Minutes **Cooked in:** 05 Minutes **How many people:** 2 Persons

Recipe Components:

- Grains and Veggies: 1 1/2 cups bulgur, 1 cup thinly sliced lacinato kale, 1/2 pound green beans, and 1-pint grape tomatoes (cut in half)
- Herbs and Spices: 1/2 cup packed basil leaves, 1/4 packed cup flat-leaf parsley, 1 garlic clove, 1 1/2 tsp kosher salt (total), and 1/4 tsp ground black pepper
- Oils and Juices: 1/4 cup lemon juice and 1/4 cup extra-virgin olive oil
- Almonds: A total of 1/4 cup plus 6 tbsp almonds (some toasted, some sliced)

Preparation Steps: The garlic cloves should be placed in the bowl of a food processor. To mince it, you may use a food processor. Put in the nuts, kale, basil, and parsley. Reduce the size of the fragments by pulsing. Throw in some pepper, salt, and lime juice. Blend the ingredients until they're as smooth as silk. Pesto is poured into bulgur. Incorporate the leftover toasted almonds, the green beans, and the tomatoes. Toss. Sprinkle some sliced almonds on top. Serve.

Nutrition Calories: 218 Kcal, Proteins: 5.6g, Fat: 14g, Carbohydrates: 18g

4.13 Turkish Scrambled Eggs
Setup Time: 08 Minutes **Cooked in:** 05 Minutes **How many people:** 4 Persons

Recipe Components:

- Veggies and Bread: 4 ripe tomatoes (diced), 4 whole grain pitas, 2 large red bell peppers (seeded and finely chopped), and 3 scallions (finely sliced)
- Dairy and Protein: 6 eggs (whisked) and 4 ozs crumbled Feta cheese
- Herbs, Spices, and Oils: 2 tbsp each of olive oil and fresh parsley (chopped), 1 tsp crushed red pepper flakes, 1/2 tsp kosher salt, and 1/4 tsp ground black pepper
- Garnish: Green olives

Preparation Steps: The oil should be heated in a pan on moderate heat. The scallions need two minutes of cooking to soften in the pan. Place the peppers inside. Stir-fry for five minutes. The tomatoes and pepper flakes should be added now. Add another five minutes of sautéing. Toss in some eggs and cheese. Shake and mix incessantly to create a scramble. The eggs need to be cooked through. Add some salt and pepper for flavor. Remove the heat source. Include the chopped parsley in the mixture. Spread olives on top. Pitas should be served on the side.

Nutrition Calories: 240 Kcal, Proteins: 12g, Fat: 14g, Carbohydrates: 19g

4.14 Swiss Chard and Red Lentil Curried Soup
Setup Time: 18 Minutes **Cooked in:** 10 Minutes **How many people:** 4 Persons

Recipe Components:

- Main Ingredients: 2 cups dried red lentils, 1 pound Swiss chard, 1 can (15 ozs) chickpeas (rinsed and drained), and 5 cups vegetable broth
- Aromatics and Veggies: 1 large onion (thinly sliced), 1 red jalapeño chili (stemmed and thinly sliced)
- Seasonings and Spices: 5 tsps curry powder, 1 tsp salt, 1/4 tsp ground cayenne pepper
- Oils and Garnish: 2 tbsp olive oil, 6 tbsp thick Greek yogurt, and 1 lime (cut into 6 wedges)

Preparation Steps: Turn on the stove to medium and add the oil to the saucepan. When the onion is tender and transparent, it is ready to be sautéed. Curry and cayenne pepper should be stirred in. Place the chard and Four cups of broth into the pot. Keep stirring at a boil till the chard is wilted, about 5 minutes. Mix in the chickpeas and beans. Reduce the level of fuel intensity. Cook the lentils at a low boil, stirring occasionally, for 18 minutes. Eliminate the source of heat or hot water. Transfer a quarter of the soup to a blender or food processor. For the sake of efficiency, of course. Return the combined liquid to the heated kettle. The remaining water and salt should be added. Stir. Get the soup nice and toasty for a few minutes on low heat. Distribute across 6 bowls. Yogurt, a lime wedge, and sliced jalapenos make a great garnish. Serve.

Nutrition Calories: 169 Kcal, Proteins: 10g, Fat: 2.82g, Carbohydrates: 26g

4.15 Orange Cardamom Quinoa with Carrots
Setup Time: 15 Minutes **Cooked in:** 0 Minutes **How many people:** 4 Persons

Recipe Components:

- Main Ingredients: 2 1/2 cups vegetable   broth, 1 pound carrots (peeled and sliced), and 1 cup quinoa (rinsed)

- Fruits and Flavor Enhancers: 2 oranges (zested and segmented), 1/3 cup golden raisins, and 1-inch piece of fresh ginger (peeled and minced)

- Spices and Seasonings: 1 tsp ground cardamom, 1/2 tsp each of freshly ground black pepper and salt

Preparation Steps: The orange zest, salt, black pepper, cardamom, raisins, ginger, carrots, quinoa, and broth go into the slow cooker. Successfully combine together and cook for 3 and a half hours. Distribute the quinoa evenly among 4 serving plates. Add a few orange segments to the top of each serving. Serve.

Nutrition Calories: 170 Kcal, Proteins: 5g, Fat: 3g, Carbohydrates: 31g

4.16 Quinoa Turmeric Power Bowl
Setup Time: 15 Minutes **Cooked in:** 30 Minutes **How many people:** 4 Persons

Recipe Components:

- 2 kale leaves (rinsed)
- 7 small yellow potatoes (slice into strips)
- 1 avocado (sliced)
- 15 ozs of drained and rinsed chickpeas
- Pepper
- 1/4 cup quinoa

- 1 tbsp. coconut oil
- 1 tsp paprika
- Salt
- 1/2 tbsp. olive oil
- 2 tsps turmeric(divided)

Preparation Steps: Turn the oven temperature up to 360 degrees Fahrenheit. Place the potato strips flat on half of the baking sheet. Coconut oil should be drizzled over the top. Add some salt, pepper, and turmeric (about a tsp's worth) for seasoning. Keep turning after 5 minutes. In a large bowl, thoroughly combine the paprika and chickpeas. Stir vigorously to combine. On the other side of the baking sheet, separate the beans from the potatoes. Set the oven timer for 25 minutes and place in oven. Put the quinoa and the liquid in a saucepan and simmer it over low to medium heat for about half an hour. Let the quinoa simmer until it's soft. Spice it up with a pinch of turmeric, some pepper, and salt. Blend well. Putting it aside to cool is a good idea. The kale benefits from a massage with olive oil. Split the leaves between 4 serving dishes. Arrange quinoa, avocado slices, and roasted veggies in separate bowls. Serve.

Nutrition Calories: 470 Kcal, Proteins: 14g, Fat: 17g, Carbohydrates: 72g

4.17 Tomato Stew with Chickpea and Kale
Setup Time: 15 Minutes **Cooked in:** 20 Minutes **How many people:** 4 Persons

Recipe Components:

- Greens and Veggies: 3/4 pound kale (stemmed and leaves coarsely chopped), 1 pound tomatoes (cored and chopped), and 1 medium onion (sectioned into eighths)
- Liquids and Beans: 1 cup vegetable stock and 2 cans (15-ounce) chickpeas (drained and rinsed)

- Aromatics and Seasonings: 6 garlic cloves (finely sliced), 1/4 tsp crushed red pepper flakes, and 1 1/4 tsp kosher salt (total)
- Oils and Proteins: 4 tbsp olive oil (to be used in portions) and 4 large eggs

Preparation Steps: In a pan over medium heat, prepare a fourth of the oil. Put a quarter of the salt in a bowl and add the onion. Cook the onions in the hot oil for ten minutes. Combine the chopped garlic and red pepper flakes. Keep cooking for another two minutes. Include the kale. Get it as soft as possible by cooking it. Add the canned tomatoes, chickpeas, and chicken stock. Prepare in ten minutes. Just add salt. Put the remaining oil in a pan and heat it over medium heat. Prepare an egg by cracking it open and cooking it till the white is done and the bottom becomes crunchy. Repeat with the remaining eggs. Create 4 bowls and equally distribute the stew. Add an egg on top. Just add salt. Serve.

Nutrition Calories: 212 Kcal, Proteins: 6.4g, Fat: 5.1g, Carbohydrates: 37g

4.18 Anti-Inflammatory Beef Meatballs
Setup Time: 10 Minutes **Cooked in:** 10 Minutes **How many people:** 4 Persons

Recipe Components:

- Main Ingredient: 2 pounds of ground beef
- Herbs and Aromatics: 1/4 cup tightly packed chopped cilantro and 5 garlic cloves (pressed)

- Spices and Zest: Zest of 1 lime, 1/2 tsp ground ginger, and 1/2 tsp sea salt

Preparation Steps: Turn on the oven and warm it to 350 degrees. Make use of parchment paper to cover a baking sheet. Combine all of the ingredients in a bowl. Never stop mixing things up. Make 12 meatballs using the mix. Place the meatballs in a single layer on a foil-lined baking sheet. Put it in the oven and pre-set the timer for 25 minutes. You may garnish the meatballs with fresh herbs and avocado slices.

Nutrition Calories: 57 Kcal, Proteins: 4g, Fat: 7g, Carbohydrates: 3g

4.19 Salmon with Veggies Sheet Pan
Setup Time: 20 Minutes **Cooked in:** 30 Minutes **How many people:** 4 Persons

Recipe Components:

Main Ingredients:
- 16 ozs bag of baby potatoes
- 16 ozs Brussels sprouts (halved)
- 4 6-ounce salmon fillets (with skin)
- 1 cup cherry tomatoes
- 1 bunch of asparagus (trimmed and split)

Aromatics and Seasonings:
- 1/2 red onion (cubed)

- 1 garlic clove (minced)
- 1 tsp fresh thyme

Dressing Ingredients:
- 3 tbsp balsamic vinegar
- 2 tbsp honey
- 2 tbsp olive oil
- 1 tbsp Dijon mustard
- 1/2 tsp sea salt

Preparation Steps: Get your oven ready for 450 F. Prepare a baking sheet with parchment paper. Mix the vinegar, garlic, honey, Dijon mustard, thyme, and salt together in a bowl to make the sauce. Maintain a healthy blend. Asparagus, red onion, Brussels sprouts, potatoes, tomatoes, olive oil, and Three tbsp. The balsamic honey combination should be combined in a separate bowl. Maintain a healthy blend. Prepare a baking sheet by spreading the veggies equally over it. Put in the oven for 10 minutes. The oven is done, so remove it. Salmon fillets should be arranged atop the veggies. It's skin-side down. Apply the remaining balsamic honey mixture to each fillet by brushing it on. The baking sheet should be returned to the oven. Put in the oven for 10 minutes. For the next four minutes, broil on high. The fillets' exposed surfaces will brown in this manner. Serve.

Nutrition Calories: 377 Kcal, Proteins: 38g, Fat: 10g, Carbohydrates: 39g

4.20 Roasted Salmon Garlic and Broccoli

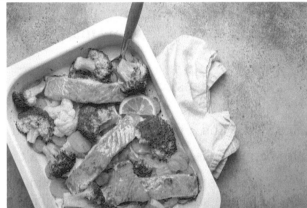

Setup Time: 25 Minutes **Cooked in:** 35 Minutes **How many people:** 4 Persons

Recipe Components:

- 1 lemon (sliced)
- 3/4 tsp sea salt (divided)
- 1 1/2 pounds salmon fillets
- 1 large broccoli head (sliced into florets)
- 2 1/2 tbsp coconut oil (melted and divided)
- 2 minced cloves fresh garlic
- Black pepper

Preparation Steps: Prepare a 450 F oven temperature. Put parchment paper on a baking sheet. Put the salmon in an even layer on the prepared baking sheet. There has to be breathing room between the various components. A tsp of olive oil should be used to finish cooking the salmon. Distribute the garlic cloves in a thin layer over the fish. Add ½ of the salt and enough pepper to taste. Place a lemon slice atop each serving of fish. Putting aside. Place the broccoli florets, remaining pepper, salt, and 1 1/2 tsps of oil in a mixing basin and toss to combine. Toss. Florets should be placed between each slice of salmon. Put the dish in the oven and set the timer for fifteen min. Parsley and lemon wedges make a lovely garnish. Serve.

Nutrition Calories: 366 Kcal, Proteins: 35g, Fat: 14g, Carbohydrates: 29g

4.21 Roasted Sweet Potatoes with Avocado Dip

Setup Time: 25 Minutes **Cooked in:** 40 Minutes **How many people:** 4 Persons

Recipe Components:

- Veggies and Fruit: 1 avocado (halved and de-seeded), 2 large sweet potatoes (cleaned and diced), and 1 lime (for juicing)
- Aromatics and Oils: 1 large garlic clove (chopped), 1 tsp + 2 tbsp olive oil
- Liquids and Seasonings: 4 tbsp water and 1/2 tsp sea salt (to be used as needed)

Preparation Steps: Turn the oven temperature up to 400 degrees F. Prepare parchment paper on a baking pan. Spread the diced potatoes out in a single layer on the prepared baking sheet. Drizzle with 2 tbsp. of olive oil. To ensure that all of the potato pieces get a coating of oil, you should turn them over. Use a third of the salt for seasoning. Cook it for 40 to 45 minutes or until it reaches the desired color in the oven. Blend the avocados with the garlic, lime juice, and the remaining half of the salt until smooth. Remove any lumps by thoroughly mixing. While stirring, gradually add the olive oil and water. Keep blending until everything is well combined. Prepare a dip to accompany the cooked potatoes and serve.

Nutrition Calories: 188 Kcal, Proteins: 3g, Fat: 13g, Carbohydrates: 20g

4.22 Chicken with Lemon and Asparagus
Setup Time: 15 Minutes **Cooked in:** 20 Minutes **How many people:** 4 Persons

Recipe Components:

- Veggies and Protein: 2 cups asparagus (chopped), 1 pound chicken breasts (boneless and skinless), and 2 lemons (sliced)
- Fats and Binders: 1/4 cup flour and 4 tbsp butter (to be used in portions)
- Seasonings: 1 tsp lemon pepper seasoning, 1/2 tsp each of salt and pepper

Preparation Steps: Lemons and Asparagus: In the same pan, over low to medium heat, melt the remaining butter. Insert the asparagus, please. The veggies should be heated until they are just soft. Put away from the heat source. Spread the lemon slices out in a single layer on the heating pan. To obtain a caramelized exterior, heat the food for several minutes on each side without stirring. Put away from the heat source. **Chicken:** To make slices that are just 3/4 of an inch thick, cut each chicken chest in half lengthwise. Put the flour, salt, and pepper into a wide, shallow dish. Combine in a harmonious manner. Sprinkle the flour mixture over each piece of chicken. Prepare the first ½ of the butter by melting it in a pan over medium heat. Place the chicken pieces within. To get a golden brown color, cook for Five minutes for each side. While cooking, season both sides of the chicken using lime pepper. Putting aside. **Assembly:** Arrange the cooked asparagus, lemon, and chicken in tiers on a serving plate. Serve.

Nutrition Calories: 250 Kcal, Proteins: 13g, Fat: 7g, Carbohydrates: 26g

4.23 Lentil Soup with Lemons
Setup Time: 15 Minutes **Cooked in:** 20 Minutes **How many people:** 8 Persons

Recipe Components:

- Veggies and Pulses: 1 1/2 cups celery (diced), 2 cups green lentils, and 1 1/2 cups carrots (chopped)
- Aromatics and Citrus: 3 cloves garlic (minced), 1 yellow onion (diced), zest of 1/2 a lemon, and 3 small lemons (for juicing)
- Liquids and Oils: 2 1/2 boxes (32 ozs each) of vegetable broth and 1 tbsp. extra-virgin olive oil
- Spices and Seasonings: 2 tsps dried turmeric, 1 tsp salt, and 4 tsps freshly grated ginger

Preparation Steps: Turn on medium heat and add oil to a Dutch oven. In a sauté pan, we saute the salt, onion, celery, and carrots for around 5 minutes. When you add the garlic and ginger, mix it thoroughly. Please give me a moment longer. In a large saucepan, combine the beans, turmeric, and chicken broth. Bring the temperature down a notch. For 45 minutes, with half the cover on, bring the soup to a boil. Blend with some fresh lime juice and zest. Mix. Add another 30 minutes to the cooking for the soup. Serve.

Nutrition Calories: 68 Kcal, Proteins: 5g, Fat: 0.5g, Carbohydrates: 12g

4.24 Shrimp Fajitas

Setup Time: 25 Minutes **Cooked in:** 25 Minutes **How many people:** 4 Persons

Recipe Components:

- Vegetables and Fruits: 1 red bell pepper (sliced thinly), 1 yellow bell pepper, 1 orange bell pepper, 1 small red onion, and lime.
- Seafood: 1 1/2 pounds of shrimp.
- Oils and Garnishes: 1 1/2 tbsp extra virgin olive oil and fresh cilantro (for garnish).
- Spices: 1 tsp kosher salt, 2 tsps chili powder, 1/2 tsp onion powder, 1/2 tsp smoked paprika, 1/2 tsp garlic powder, 1/2 tsp ground cumin, and freshly ground pepper.
- Others: Warmed Tortillas.

Preparation Steps: The oven should be preheated at 450 degrees F. Spray cooking spray onto a baking sheet. Put the shrimp, peppers, onions, spices, olive oil, and salt into a large mixing bowl. Make sure to give it a good toss. Distribute them in a single layer on the baking sheet. Put in oven and bake for 10 min. Go ahead and turn the oven to broil. To finish cooking the fajita, wait 2 minutes. Lime juice should be squeezed over the fajita. Use cilantro as a garnish. Put on heated tortillas and serve.

Nutrition Calories: 241 Kcal, Proteins: 14g, Fat: 10g, Carbohydrates: 25g

3.25 Mediterranean One Pan Cod

Setup Time: 15 Minutes **Cooked in:** 20 Minutes **How many people:** 4 Persons

Recipe Components:

- Vegetables: 2 cups fennel (sliced), 2 cups kale (shredded), 1 cup fresh tomatoes (diced), 1 small onion (sliced).

- Proteins: 1 pound cod (quartered).

- Canned Goods: 1 can (14.5 ozs) diced tomato.

- Oils and Liquids: 2 tbsp olive oil, 1/2 cup water.

- Herbs, Spices, and Seasonings: 3 large cloves of garlic (chopped), pinch of red pepper (crushed), 1 tsp orange zest, 1/2 tsp dried oregano, 1/4 tsp black pepper, 1/4 tsp fennel seeds, 1/8 tsp salt.

- Other Ingredients: 1 cup oil-cured black olives.

Garnish:

- Orange zest
- Fresh oregano
- Fennel fronds
- Olive oil

Preparation Steps: In a pan, warm the olive oil over medium heat. It's recommended to saute fennel, onion, and garlic together for 8 minutes. Salt and pepper are optional. Add the water, fresh tomatoes, canned tomatoes, and kale. Just increase the cooking time by 12 minutes. Season with oregano, black pepper, and olives, then mix everything together. Toss the fish with a mixture of pepper, fennel seeds, salt, and lemon or lime juice. Place the fish fillets in the tomato sauce. Tightly cover the skillet. Ten minutes at a low simmer. Garnish. Serve.

Nutrition Calories: 333 Kcal, Proteins: 43g, Fat: 10g, Carbohydrates: 19g

4.26 Garlic Tomato Basil Chicken

Setup Time: 20 Minutes **Cooked in:** 15 Minutes **How many people:** 4 Persons

Recipe Components:

- Proteins: 1 pound of chicken breasts (boneless and skinless).
- Vegetables: 4 medium zucchini (spiralized), 1/2 yellow onion (diced).
- Herbs and Spices: 1 cup fresh basil (loosely packed and cut into ribbons), 3 garlic cloves (minced), 1/4 tsp red pepper flakes (crushed).
- Canned Goods: 14.5 oz can of chopped tomatoes.
- Oils and Seasonings: 2 tbsp olive oil (divided), salt, and pepper.

Preparation Steps: Use plastic wrap to enclose each chicken breast. Beat them to a uniform thickness of one inch. Tear open each chicken breast. Season with salt and pepper to taste. Heat a pan with a teaspoon of olive oil on a medium heat. Cook the chicken breasts in a skillet. They need to be cooked thoroughly by browning in a pan. In the same pan, warm the remaining olive oil over low heat. The onion should be cooked for approximately 5 minutes before the garlic is added. Continue to stir-fry for another minute. Combine the tomatoes and basil and stir to combine. Crush some red pepper, grind some black pepper, and sprinkle some salt on it, to taste. Put it on low heat and mix it every so often for 10 minutes. Mix in the chicken breasts and zoodles. Allow to heat slowly for a couple of moments. Serve.

Nutrition Calories: 686 Kcal, Proteins: 34g, Fat: 40g, Carbohydrates: 46g

4.27 Asian Garlic Noodles

Setup Time: 05 Minutes **Cooked in:** 10 Minutes **How many people:** 4 Persons

Recipe Components:

Noodles:

- 1 small red bell pepper (minced)
- 1 large spaghetti squash
- 1/2 cup fresh cilantro (diced)
- 1/2 large carrot (julienne cut)
- 1/4 cup roasted cashews (chopped)
- 1/2 medium zucchini (julienne cut)

Sauce:

- 6 garlic cloves
- 6 large Medjool dates (pitted)
- 2 tbsp fish sauce
- 1/4 cup coconut milk (full fat)
- 2 tbsp red curry paste
- 2/3 cup coconut aminos
- 2 tbsp fresh ginger (grated)

Preparation Steps: Your microwave oven has to be preheated to 425 degrees F. Prepare the spaghetti squash by slicing it in half lengthwise. Use a scraper to get rid of the pulp. Place the spaghetti squash on a baking pan cut side up. The affected region should be rubbed with olive oil. Prepare a 30-minute timer for the oven. You may get a noodle-like texture by scraping the meat with a fork. Put all the sauce ingredients into a blender and mix until smooth. Puree. Throw all the noodle-making stuff into a bowl and mix it together. Cover the noodles with the sauce. Combine in a harmonious manner. Serve.

Nutrition Calories: 426 Kcal, Proteins: 30g, Fat: 7g, Carbohydrates: 62g

4.28 Shrimp Garlic Zoodles

Setup Time: 15 Minutes **Cooked in:** 05 Minutes **How many people:** 4 Persons

Recipe Components:

- Vegetables & Fruits: 2 medium zucchini, zest and juice of 1 lemon.
- Seafood: 3/4 pounds medium shrimp.
- Aromatics: 4 cloves garlic (minced).
- Oils & Seasonings: 1 tbsp. olive oil, salt, pepper, and red pepper flakes.
- Herbs: Fresh parsley (chopped).

Preparation Steps: Cook the zoodles in a spiralizer set to medium. Putting aside. Over low to medium heat, combine the olive oil, lime juice, and lime zest. The shrimp has to be put in and mixed around. You should still leave it in the oven for a few more minutes. Add the minced garlic and crushed red pepper to a bowl and mix well. Just one more minute, please. Prepare the zucchini noodles. To get a medium-rare doneness, turn the meat for three minutes. Salt and pepper are optional. Sprinkle some chopped parsley on top. Serve.

Nutrition Calories: 286 Kcal, Proteins: 27g, Fat: 5.7g, Carbohydrates: 8.1g

4.29 Cauliflower Grits and Shrimp

Setup Time: 15 Minutes **Cooked in:** 05 Minutes **How many people:** 4 Persons

Recipe Components:

Cauliflower Grits:

- 1 large clove of garlic (chopped)
- 1 bag (12 ozs) of frozen cauliflower
- Salt
- 2 tbsp butter

Shrimp:

- 3 tbsp Cajun seasoning (no salt)
- 1 pound large shrimp (peeled and deveined)
- 2 tbsp butter
- Salt

Preparation Steps: The cauliflower and the garlic should be steamed together in a pot. Waiting to be steamed till soft. (The piping hot liquid should not be thrown away). Combine the steamed cauliflower, garlic, and butter in a food processor and pulse until smooth. During the course of processing, the consistency may be modified as needed. To adjust the consistency, just add more hot water or salt and stir. Leaving aside. Mix all of the Cajun spices together. The shrimp need more seasoning than just a sprinkle. Season with salt. In a pan, melt the butter over medium heat. Throw in some shrimp. The beef should be cooked to an internal temperature of 160 degrees Fahrenheit. The grits and cauliflower should be split between two dishes. Place the shrimp on top once they have been cooked. When serving, transfer the gravy from the pan to the bowls. Serve.

Nutrition Calories: 350 Kcal, Proteins: 37g, Fat: 16g, Carbohydrates: 21g

4.30 Green Curry

Setup Time: 20 Minutes **Cooked in:** 15 Minutes **How many people:** 4 Persons

Recipe Components:

- 12 ozs tofu (firm)
- 3 cups broccoli florets
- A swish of olive oil
- 3 cans (14 ozs) of coconut milk

- 2 sweet potatoes (peeled and cubed)
- 4 tbsp green curry paste
- A sprinkle of salt

Garnish:

- Fresh cilantro (chopped)
- Fish sauce

- Golden raisins
- Brown sugar

Preparation Steps: Use towels to rinse the tofu. Cube the tofu and set it aside. Put the olive oil in a pan and warm it over moderate heat. Toss the tofu in the pan. Put some salt on it. Cook the tofu in hot oil for fifteen min, occasionally turning until it is golden brown all over. Putting aside. Mix the curry paste, coconut milk, and sweet potatoes in the same saucepan and heat over medium. Hold at a low boil for ten min. Add the broccoli and tofu to the pan. Simmer for another 5 minutes. Flourish. Serve.

Nutrition Calories: 328 Kcal, Proteins: 24g, Fat: 20g, Carbohydrates: 17g

CHAPTER 5: Anti-Inflammatory Dinner Recipes

5.1 Stir-Fried Snap Pea and Chicken

Setup Time: 20 Minutes **Cooked in:** 15 Minutes **How many people:** 4 Persons

Recipe Components:

- Vegetables and Herbs: 2 1/2 cups sweet peas, 1 red bell pepper, 1 bunch of scallions, and 3 tbsp fresh cilantro.

- Protein: 1 1/4 cups of skinless, boneless, and thinly sliced chicken breast.

- Condiments and Oils: 3 tbsp soy sauce, 2 tbsp of each vegetable oil and rice vinegar, and 2 tsp Sriracha.

- Seasonings: Salt, ground black pepper, and 2 garlic cloves.

- Garnish: 2 tbsp sesame seeds (+ extra for garnishing).

Preparation Steps: First, clean the shallot and garlic and then place them in the pan with the addition of a drizzle of oil. After cooking them for about 60 seconds, you are ready to add the peas and pepper and continue cooking for a few minutes. After the time indicated above, insert the chicken and cook everything for another 5 minutes. While cooking, place the rice vinegar, sesame seeds, soy sauce, and Sriracha in a bowl and mix everything well. Cook the mixture for 2 minutes and add the chopped coriander. When everything is ready, you can serve.

Nutrition Calories: 261 Kcal, Proteins: 29g, Fat: 10g, Carbohydrates: 14g

5.2 Turkey Chili with Avocado

Setup Time: 25 Minutes **Cooked in:** 22 Minutes **How many people:** 8 Persons

Recipe Components:

- Proteins and Legumes: 1 pound ground turkey, 1 can (15 ozs) of white beans.
- Liquids: 4 cups chicken broth, 2 tbsp extra-virgin olive oil.

- Vegetables and Condiments: 1 large white onion (diced), 1 can (15 ozs) of corn kernels, 1 avocado (diced), 4 garlic cloves (minced).
- Seasonings: 2 tsps ground cumin, 1 tsp ground coriander, 1 tsp cayenne pepper, salt, and freshly ground black pepper.

Preparation Steps: After cleaning the onion with a knife, please place it in a pan and cook for 8 minutes, remembering to use a drizzle of oil. Now, you can add the garlic. Keep the heat low for another minute of sautéing. Place the turkey inside. To ensure thorough cooking, set the timer for 7 minutes. Spice it up with cayenne pepper, cumin, coriander, pepper and salt. Mixed. Leave it on the heat for a few minutes. Add the broth to the pot. The ingredients should be left to simmer for 35 minutes. Prepare the corn and beans. Keep at a low boil for another 3 minutes. Add some chopped avocado on top of each plate. Serve.

Nutrition Calories: 686 Kcal, Proteins: 47g, Fat: 46g, Carbohydrates: 14g

5.3 Grecian-Style Turkey Burgers with Tzatziki

Setup Time: 22 Minutes **Cooked in:** 20 Minutes **How many people:** 4 Persons

Recipe Components:

- Meat & Vegetables: 1 pound ground turkey, 1 sweet onion (minced), and 2 garlic cloves (minced).
- Binders & Seasonings: 3/4 cup bread crumbs, 1 egg, 1/2 tsp dried oregano, 1/4 tsp red-pepper flakes, salt, and freshly ground black pepper.
- Herbs & Oil: 1/2 cup fresh parsley (chopped) and 1 tbsp. extra-virgin olive oil.

Tzatziki Sauce:

- Base & Flavorings: 1 cup Greek yogurt, 1/2 European cucumber (diced), and 1 pinch of garlic powder.
- Liquids & Herbs: 1/4 cup fresh parsley (chopped), 2 tbsp lemon juice, and 1 tbsp. extra-virgin olive oil.
- Seasonings: Salt and freshly ground black pepper.

Toppings:

- Fresh Produce & Bread: 2 tomatoes (sliced), 1/2 red onion (sliced), 8 Boston lettuce leaves, and 4 whole-wheat hamburger buns.

Preparation Steps: Burgers: Remove the peel from the onion and garlic, place them in a pan previously greased with a drizzle of oil, and cook for a few minutes. Maintain the low heat for one more minute of sauteing. Putting aside. Combine the turkey, oregano, pepper flakes, parsley, cooled onion, and egg in a large mixing basin. Combine in a harmonious manner. Add the bread crumbs, seasoning, and pepper. Combine in a harmonious manner. Turn the oven temperature up to 350 degrees F. Make 4 burgers out of the turkey mixture. Put some cooking spray in a skillet that can go from the stovetop to the oven and heat it over medium. Place the burger inside. Brown the meat by searing it for 5 minutes on each side. You should bake the skillet. The burgers need to be baked for 17 minutes. **Tzatziki Sauce:** To make your own sauce, you need to mix garlic powder, olive oil, lime juice, yogurt and cucumber. When the mixture is smooth, season with salt and pepper to taste and finish with a pinch of parsley.

Nutrition Calories: 350 Kcal, Proteins: 54g, Fat: 7g, Carbohydrates: 10g

5.4 Fried Rice with Pineapple

Setup Time: 10 Minutes **Cooked in:** 15 Minutes **How many people:** 3 Persons

Recipe Components:

- Grains and Vegetables: 3 cups cooked brown rice, 2 peeled and grated carrots, 1 diced onion, 2 sliced green onions.
- Fruits and Proteins: 2 cups pineapple (diced), 1/2 cup ham (diced).
- Frozen Ingredients: 1/2 cup frozen corn, 1/2 cup frozen peas.

- Oils and Condiments: 3 tbsp soy sauce, 1 tbsp. sesame oil, 2 tbsp olive oil.
- Aromatics and Spices: 2 minced cloves garlic, 1/2 tsp ginger powder, 1/4 tsp white pepper.

Preparation Steps: The first thing to do is to take a pan and put it on the heat. Inside, you must put the already cleaned garlic and onion and cook them for a few minutes. While cooking, prepare the mixture made of soy sauce, sesame oil, ginger powder, and white ginger powder.

When the contents of the pan are golden, you can add the vegetables and continue the cooking phase until they are soft. Finally, add the rice mixture, pineapple, ham, green onions, and soy sauce to the pan. Continue stirring for a few minutes while the food cooks. When everything is ready, you can serve.

Nutrition Calories: 179 Kcal, Proteins: 3g, Fat: 5g, Carbohydrates: 30g

5.5 Ratatouille

Setup Time: 10 Minutes **Cooked in:** 15 Minutes **How many people:** 5 Persons

Recipe Components:

- 1 medium red onion (thickly sliced)
- 1 small eggplant
- 1 cup tomato sauce
- 2 small red bell peppers (halved)
- 2 medium summer squash
- Salt
- 2 medium zucchini
- 3 medium tomatoes
- 2 sprigs oregano
- 2 garlic cloves (smashed)
- Black pepper to season
- 2 tbsp thyme leaves
- 5 tbsp olive oil

Preparation Steps: While you prepare the ingredients, set the oven to 375° and let it heat up. Clean the garlic and place it in a baking dish with a drizzle of oil oregano and cook for a few minutes, then remove them. Place the vegetables in the baking dish and the tomato sauce at the base. Add the remaining sauce on top. Add the aromas to give flavor, and cook everything for about half an hour. Check occasionally and serve when cooked.

Nutrition Calories: 127 Kcal, Proteins: 2.1g, Fat: 7.1g, Carbohydrates: 16g

5.6 Eggs with Tomatoes and Asparagus

Setup Time: 10 Minutes **Cooked in:** 10 Minutes **How many people:** 4 Persons

Recipe Components:

- 2 pounds asparagus
- 1-pint cherry tomatoes
- 4 eggs
- Salt
- 2 tbsp olive oil
- 2 tsps fresh thyme (chopped)
- Pepper

Preparation Steps: Place the asparagus and the tomato in a pan greased with a drizzle of oil. Season the mixture with the spices. Once the oven you have turned on has reached a temperature of 400°F, you can cook the mixture for 12 minutes. When the vegetables are cooked, prepare the eggs and make the omelet. Serve when cooked.

Nutrition Calories: 290 Kcal, Proteins: 13g, Fat: 17g, Carbohydrates: 21g

5.7 Turmeric, Carrot, and Ginger Soup

Setup Time: 10 Minutes **Cooked in:** 10 Minutes **How many people:** 4 Persons

Recipe Components:

- 3 carrots (diced)
- 4 cups vegetable stock
- Canned coconut milk (for topping)
- 3 cloves garlic (minced)
- 1-inch fresh ginger (finely grated)
- 2 inches of fresh turmeric (finely grated)
- 1 white onion (diced)
- Black sesame seeds (for topping)
- 1 tbsp. lemon juice

Preparation Steps: Put some olive oil in a saucepan and cook it over medium heat. Caramelize the onion in a skillet. Prepare the dish by adding the spices. Keep cooking for another minute. Prepare by adding carrots. To prepare, you will need to spend two minutes cooking. Incorporate the vegetable stock. Maintain a low boil for 25 minutes. Use a stick blender to purée the soup. Prepare the dish by adding lemon juice. Stir. To serve, stir with some coconut milk and sprinkle with black sesame seeds.

Nutrition Calories: 103 Kcal, Proteins: 2g, Fat: 3g, Carbohydrates: 18g

5.8 Bulgur and Sweet Potato Salad
Setup Time: 15 Minutes **Cooked in:** 40 Minutes **How many people:** 4 Persons

Recipe Components:

- Main Ingredients: 1 1/4 cups bulgur wheat, 2 medium sweet potatoes.
- Fresh Produce and Herbs: 1 cup parsley, 1/2 cup mint, 1/4 cup red onion, 2 tbsp orange zest.
- Liquids and Oils: 1/4 cup olive oil, 1/4 cup freshly squeezed orange juice, 2 tbsp lemon juice, 1 tbsp. avocado oil, 1 tbsp. red wine vinegar.
- Flavor Enhancers: 2 tsps maple syrup, 1 small clove of garlic (grated).
- Seasonings: coarse salt, 1/2 tsp, salt freshly ground black pepper, black pepper.

Preparation Steps: Peel the potatoes and then soak them in the avocado oil and maple syrup. While you prepare this mixture, raise the oven temperature to 450°F. Put the spices in the mixture created to improve the flavor, and when ready, put it in a baking pan. Cook with the roast mode active for approximately 40 minutes. During cooking, prepare a pot with water and put it on the heat until it boils. Place the cooked mixture in the oven and continue cooking at a low temperature. When cooked, after about 8/10 minutes, put the lid on and let it rest. In a bowl, prepare the sauce by adding garlic, vinegar, salt, citrus juices, and pepper. When well mixed, add the remaining ingredients, and when everything is ready and tasty, serve and enjoy it.

Nutrition Calories: 103 Kcal, Proteins: 2g, Fat: 3g, Carbohydrates: 18g

5.9 Salmon Roast with Romaine and Potatoes
Setup Time: 15 Minutes **Cooked in:** 30 Minutes **How many people:** 4 Persons

Recipe Components:

- 2 hearts of romaine lettuce (cut in half)
- 1 pound of baby potatoes (rinsed)
- 4 (6-ounce) salmon fillets
- 1 tbsp. butter (melted)
- 4 tbsp olive oil (divided)
- 1 tsp lemon juice
- Freshly ground black pepper
- 1/4 tsp paprika

- Salt

Preparation Steps: Check that you have all the ingredients necessary to carry out the recipe and start by turning on the oven and setting it so that its temperature reaches 450° quickly. Once this first step has been done, serve a baking tray for which you will place the potatoes, which I have oiled with a drizzle of olive oil, and place them in the hot oven before moving on to the cooking phase. In the meantime, take the lettuce leaves and pass them with oil, lemon juice, and spices to give a tasty punch to the dish. Place the salmon fillets on the leaves and rub melted butter on each of them. Cook everything in the oven for about 8 minutes, and when ready, serve.

Nutrition Calories: 147 Kcal, Proteins: 0g, Fat: 4g, Carbohydrates: 1g

5.10 Bean Bolognese
Setup Time: 15 Minutes **Cooked in:** 30 Minutes **How many people:** 4 Persons

Recipe Components:

- 14 oz white beans
- 2 ready to use carrots
- 1 medium onion
- 28 oz crushed tomatoes
- 2 of each cloves of garlic and celery stalks

Preparation Steps: Put everything into a slow cooker. Put it in the oven and let it there for 6 hours. Serve.

Nutrition Calories: 442 Kcal, Proteins: 17g, Fat: 11g, Carbohydrates: 68g

5.11 Peppers Stuffed with Sweet Potato and Turkey
Setup Time: 15 Minutes **Cooked in:** 20 Minutes **How many people:** 4 Persons

Recipe Components:

- 1 2/3 cups sweet potatoes (diced)
- 2 cups ground turkey
- 1/2 cup tomato sauce
- 2 large bell peppers (cut in half)
- 1/2 cup onions (diced)
- 1 tbsp. extra-virgin olive oil
- Pepper
- 2 cloves garlic (minced)
- Fresh parsley (for garnishing)
- Salt

Preparation Steps: To cook the turkey, you will need to prepare a baking tray with a drizzle of oil and place the meat on it. Also, add an already-cleaned clove of garlic and put it in the oven. The oven must have a temperature of 350°. After the first 7 minutes of cooking, add the potatoes, which, in the meantime, you will have peeled and prepared, and the onions. After a few minutes of cooking, add the seasonings and the tomato. When the mixture is ready, chop it up and create a mush that I would put inside the peppers. At this point, cook the peppers in the oven, and when ready, enjoy them with your family.

Nutrition Calories: 324 Kcal, Proteins: 25g, Fat: 13g, Carbohydrates: 26g

5.12 Turkey Meatballs

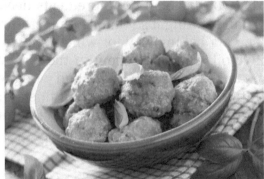

Setup Time: 10 Minutes **Cooked in:** 30 Minutes **How many people:** 4 Persons

Recipe Components:

- 1/2 cup Grated Parmesan cheese
- 1 pound ground turkey
- 1/2 cup fresh breadcrumbs (whole wheat)
- 2-3 tbsp of water
- 1 large egg (beaten)
- 1 tbsp. fresh parsley
- 1/2 tbsp. of basil and oregano
- Pinch of fresh nutmeg

Preparation Steps: To prepare tasty meatballs, you will need to put the following ingredients from the list above in a large enough bowl: breadcrumbs, beaten egg, grated cheese, chopped turkey, and a little water. Mix the first time and season with the aromatic herbs, salt, nutmeg, and a pinch of pepper. Continue mixing until you create a homogeneous mixture that does not fall apart. Make about 30 meatballs and place them in a pan with a drizzle of olive oil. Before starting the preparation, heat the oven and set it so that the internal temperature is 350°. When both the oven and the mixture and the meatballs are ready, you will have to cook them for half an hour. Enjoy them with your guests.

Nutrition Calories: 140 Kcal, Proteins: 14g, Fat: 9g, Carbohydrates: 5g

5.13 Chicken Chili and White Beans

Setup Time: 15 Minutes **Cooked in:** 20 Minutes **How many people:** 4 Persons

Recipe Components:

- Meats and Liquids: 2 cups shredded cooked chicken breast, 3 cups chicken stock, 1 cup nut milk.
- Vegetables: 1 cup chopped Brussels sprouts, 1 chopped leek, 1 chopped small onion, 1 seeded and diced jalapeño pepper, 1 large peeled and chopped white potato.
- Beans and Oils: 1 can (15-ounce) small white beans, 2 tbsp olive oil.
- Spices and Herbs: 1 tbsp. ground cumin, 2 minced garlic cloves, 1 tsp dried oregano, a pinch of crushed red pepper flakes.

Garnish:

- Tortilla chips
- Jalapeño slices
- Shredded cheese
- Hot sauce

Preparation Steps: Olive oil should be heated over medium heat in a saucepan.

Saute the onion and jalapeno, and leak for about 5 minutes. Combine the minced garlic and spices. Get set to wait for one minute. Throw in some chicken, stock, white beans, Brussels sprouts, and potatoes. Stir. For twenty minutes, keep covered and at a low simmer. Bring milk, just in case! Stir. Get set to wait for one minute. Add the garnishes, and it's ready to serve.

Nutrition Calories: 502 Kcal, Proteins: 45g, Fat: 12g, Carbohydrates: 58g

5.14 Cauliflower Rice and Salmon Bowl
Setup Time: 15 Minutes **Cooked in:** 20 Minutes **How many people:** 4 Persons

Recipe Components:

- 1/2 head cauliflower (riced)
- 2 salmon fillets
- 1 bunch kale (shredded)
- 1 tsp curry powder

- 3 tbsp olive oil
- 12 Brussels sprouts (halved)
- Himalayan salt

Marinade:

- Sauce Components: 1/4 cup tamari sauce, 1 tsp Dijon mustard, 1 tsp maple syrup.

- Oil and Seeds: 1 tsp sesame oil, 1 tbsp. sesame seeds.

Preparation Steps: Get the oven ready at 350 degrees. Prepare parchment paper on a baking pan. The Brussels sprouts should be placed on the prepared baking sheet. Put a spoonful of olive oil on it and coat it well. Prepare by adding salt. Cook at 400° for 20 minutes. Combine the marinade's components in a basin. Mix and harmonize the ingredients. Instead of Brussels sprouts, swap up some salmon fillets for the baking dish. The marinade should be sprinkled on top of the fillets. Bake at 400° for 15 minutes. In a small saucepan, heat 1 tsp of olive oil over low to medium heat. You should sauté the greens for three minutes. For the time being, set aside. Reduce the heat to medium and re-use the same pan to add the rest of the olive oil. The curry powder, cauliflower rice, and salt should be added now. Stir-fry for three minutes. Split the salmon and brussels sprouts between two plates. To finish, sprinkle some kale and cauliflower rice over the top. Serve.

Nutrition Calories: 502 Kcal, Proteins: 45g, Fat: 12g, Carbohydrates: 58g

5.15 Harissa and Chicken Tenders
Setup Time: 15 Minutes **Cooked in:** 15 Minutes **How many people:** 6 Persons

Recipe Components:

- 1/4 cup plain Greek yogurt
- 2 tbsp harissa paste

- 24 pieces of chicken tenders
- 1/4 cup dry white wine

Preparation Steps: Place the yogurt, wine, and harissa in a bowl. Combine everything well. Chicken tenders should be inserted. Apply the marinade to the tenders. Cover. Put the marinade into the fridge and let it sit for at least two hours. Grills should be preheated. The chicken strips need to be drained. Allow any surplus liquid to drain. Cook the tenders on the grill for 5 minutes total. You may make a sandwich out of the tenders. Add your favorite fresh herbs and sliced vegetables on top.

Nutrition Calories: 800 Kcal, Proteins: 51g, Fat: 37g, Carbohydrates: 62g

5.16 Chinese Chicken Salad

Setup Time: 15 Minutes **Cooked in:** 10 Minutes **How many people:** 4 Persons

Recipe Components:

Dressing:

- 1/2 cup vegetable oil
- 1/4 cup unseasoned rice wine vinegar
- A pinch of salt to season the dish
- 1 tbsp. low-sodium soy sauce, and Dijon mustard
- 1 tsp sesame oil.
- garlic cloves
- 1/4-inch ready-to-use ginger

Salad:

- Proteins and Vegetables: 4 cups shredded green cabbage, 2 shredded cooked chicken breasts, 1 cup shredded red cabbage, 1 small carrot (cut into thin strips), 4 scallions (thinly sliced).
- Beans and Herbs: 1/4 cup cooked edamame, 1/2 cup chopped cilantro leaves, 2 tbsp chopped mint leaves.
- Garnish: Wonton strips.

Preparation Steps: All the ingredients in the list of dressing above must be combined and then blended together. In a salad bowl, place all the ingredients intended for its creation and season. Add wonton strips and enjoy.

Nutrition Calories: 97 Kcal, Proteins: 8.2g, Fat: 3g, Carbohydrates: 9g

5.17 Baked Cauliflower Buffalo

Setup Time: 15 Minutes **Cooked in:** 10 Minutes **How many people:** 4 Persons

Recipe Components:

- 1/4 cup water
- 1/2 cup hot sauce
- 1/4 cup banana flour
- 2 tbsp butter (melted)
- 1 medium cauliflower (bite-sized)
- Pinch of pepper
- Ranch dressing (for serving)
- Pinch of salt

Preparation Steps: First, set the oven temperature to 425 degrees F. Cover a baking tray with foil. Water, pepper, flour, and salt should be combined in a bowl. Combine everything well. Cauliflower should be included. Mix well by tossing. Arrange the coated cauliflower in an even layer on the prepared baking sheet. Put in the oven for fifteen min. Midway through cooked, turn the cauliflower over. The butter and spicy sauce should be combined in a separate bowl. Combine everything well. Coat the cauliflower with the sauce. Add another 20 minutes of baking time. Toss with ranch dressing and serve.

Nutrition Calories: 52 Kcal, Proteins: 2g, Fat: 2g, Carbohydrates: 6.4g

5.18 Kale and Sweet Potato Tostadas

Setup Time: 15 Minutes **Cooked in:** 10 Minutes **How many people:** 4 Persons

Recipe Components:

- 2 medium sweet potatoes (cleaned and chopped)
- 8 stems of kale (roughly chopped)
- 12 Brussels sprouts (finely chopped)
- 1 tbsp. lime juice
- 2 tbsp olive oil
- 1 tbsp. olive oil
- Pinch of salt
- 1 tsp honey
- Corn tortillas
- Pinch of cayenne pepper
- Toasted coconut
- Fresh mint (chopped)
- Yogurt

Preparation Steps: Turn the oven temperature up to 400 degrees F. Using foil, effective style baking sheets. The sweet potatoes should be placed on a baking pan that has been lined. Use olive oil as a finishing touch. Spike it up with some cayenne pepper. Just toss it on the coat. The greens should go on the second baking sheet that has been prepared in the same way. Dress with a drizzle of olive oil. Prepare by adding salt. Just toss it on the coat. Fire up the oven with both baking trays inside. For just around 10 minutes, the kale may be roasted. For Forty minutes, roast the sweet potatoes. Combine the Brussels sprouts, honey, and lime juice in a bowl. Mix well by tossing. Corn tortillas may be piled high on a sheet of aluminum foil. Put it in a preheated 3-minute toasting cycle in the oven. Wrap the sweet potato and greens in a tortilla. Sprinkle some toasted coconut, mint, yogurt, and Brussels sprouts on top. Serve.

Nutrition Calories: 190 Kcal, Proteins: 5g, Fat: 8g, Carbohydrates: 25g

CHAPTER 6: Anti-Inflammatory Snack Recipes

6.1 Spicy Tuna Rolls
Setup Time: 15 Minutes **Cooked in:** 10 Minutes **How many people:** 4 Persons

Recipe Components:

- 1 medium cucumber
- 1 pouch Yellowfin Tuna
- 1/16 tsp ground cayenne
- 2 avocado slices (cut into 6 pieces in total)
- 1/8 tsp pepper
- 1 tsp hot sauce
- 1/8 tsp salt

Preparation Steps: Cut the cucumber into thin, long slices. Cucumbers used for slicing must be seedless. Generate a total of six servings. Roll the slices in paper towels to dry them. Combine the tuna, pepper, cayenne, salt, and spicy sauce in a bowl. Combine everything well. Top the cucumber rounds with the tuna spread. Avoid crowding the edges. The dish would benefit from one avocado slice. Carefully roll the cucumber. Insert toothpicks into each roll to keep it together. Serve.

Nutrition Calories: 190 Kcal, Proteins: 6g, Fat: 6g, Carbohydrates: 24g

6.2 Turmeric Gummies

Setup Time: 15 Minutes **Cooked in:** 20 Minutes **How many people:** 6 Persons

Recipe Components:

- 8 tbsp gelatin powder (unflavored)
- 3 1/2 cups of water
- 6 tbsp maple syrup
- Pinch of ground pepper
- 1 tsp ground turmeric

Preparation Steps: Combine the water, turmeric, and maple syrup in a saucepan and boil over medium. Stir constantly and let cook for 5 minutes. Shut off the furnace. Blend with some gelatin powder. Combine everything well. Bring the temperature up to maximum. In order to mix the gelatin powder, stir the contents of the saucepan vigorously. Fill molds made of silicon with the mixture. Cover. Put in the refrigerator and chill for at least four hours. Cut them up into manageable gummy chunks. Serve.

Nutrition Calories: 22 Kcal, Proteins: 0g, Fat: 0g, Carbohydrates: 5.2g

6.3 Ginger-Cinnamon Mixed Nuts
Setup Time: 10 Minutes **Cooked in:** 15 Minutes **How many people:** 4 Persons

Recipe Components:

- 2 large egg whites
- Coconut oil spray
- 2 cups mixed nuts
- 1 tsp fresh ginger (grated)
- 1/2 tsp fine sea salt
- 1/2 tsp ground Vietnamese cinnamon

Preparation Steps: Get the oven ready at 250 degrees F. Place the egg whites in a large mixing dish. Mix with a mixer until foamy. Mix in the salt, ginger, and cinnamon. Combine all of the ingredients by whipping them together. Add the roasted and salted mixed nuts. The coating may be achieved with a good mix. Spray coconut oil onto a sheet of parchment paper. Prepare a baking sheet with parchment paper. Create a flat layer of nuts on the baking sheet. Put it in the oven and set the timer for 40 minutes. Halfway through, flip the baking sheet. It's best to wait until the nuts have cooled and hardened. Split them apart and use the pieces in various ways. Serve.

Nutrition Calories: 173 Kcal, Proteins: 5g, Fat: 16g, Carbohydrates: 6g

6.4 Ginger Date Almond Bars

Setup Time: 5 Minutes **Cooked in:** 15 Minutes **How many people:** 4 Persons

Recipe Components:

- 1 tsp ground ginger
- 1/4 cup almond milk
- 1 cup almond flour
- 3/4 cup dates

Preparation Steps: Get the oven ready at 350 degrees. Mix the dates and almond milk in a blender. Put everything in a blender and whir it for 5 minutes until it becomes a paste. Add the ground almonds and ginger. Put in other ingredients and blend for three more minutes. Place the ingredients in a casserole. Hold off till it cools. Break up into eight bars. Serve.

Nutrition Calories: 270 Kcal, Proteins: 10g, Fat: 16g, Carbohydrates: 24g

6.5 Coffee Cacao Protein Bars

Setup Time: 5 Minutes **Cooked in:** 20 Minutes **How many people:** 8 Persons

Recipe Components:

- 18 large Medjool dates (pitted)
- 2 cups mixed nuts
- 1 cup egg white protein powder
- 3 tbsp instant coffee powder
- 1/4 cup cacao powder
- 1/4 cup cacao nibs
- 5 tbsp water

Preparation Steps: Put parchment paper in an 8x8-inch square baking dish. Combine the coffee, egg white protein powder, cacao powder, and almonds in a food processor. The nuts should be processed until they are in very minute bits. Include the dates. Combining procedure. Add water, 1 tbsp. at a time, while processing, until a sticky consistency is reached. You need to take the processor's S-blade out. Chop up the cacao nibs and add them to the mixture. Put the liquid into the prepared square baking dish. Use a roller to make the mixture uniformly flat. Keep cold for at least 60 minutes. Separate into 16 pieces. Serve.

Nutrition Calories: 246 Kcal, Proteins: 12g, Fat: 12g, Carbohydrates: 19g

30-Day Anti-Inflammatory Meal Plan

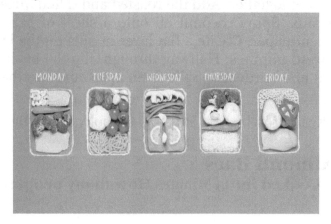

Day 1

Breakfast: Chia Seed and Milk Pudding

Lunch: Buddha Bowl with Avocado, Wild Rice, Kale, and Orange

Dinner: Stir-Fried Snap Pea and Chicken

Snack: Spicy Tuna Rolls

Day 2

Breakfast: Scrambled Eggs with Turmeric

Lunch: Avocado Chickpea Salad Sandwich

Dinner: Turkey Chili with Avocado

Snack: Turmeric Gummies

Day 3

Breakfast: Protein-Rich Turmeric Donuts

Lunch: Spiced Lentil Soup

Dinner: Grecian-Style Turkey Burgers with Tzatziki

Snack: Ginger-Cinnamon Mixed Nuts

Day 4

Breakfast: Cranberry and Sweet Potato Bars

Lunch: Red Lentil Pasta with Tomato

Dinner: Fried Rice with Pineapple

Snack: Ginger Date Almond Bars

Day 5

Breakfast: Nutty Choco-Nana Pancakes

Lunch: Tuna Mediterranean Salad

Dinner: Ratatouille

Snack: Coffee Cacao Protein Bars

Day 6

Breakfast: Blueberry Avocado Chocolate Muffins

Lunch: Chicken and Greek Salad Wrap

Dinner: Eggs with Tomatoes and Asparagus

Snack: Spicy Tuna Rolls

Day 7

Breakfast: Tropical Smoothie Bowl

Lunch: Cauliflower and Chickpea

Coconut Curry

Dinner: Turmeric, Carrot, and Ginger Soup

Snack: Turmeric Gummies

Day 8

Breakfast: Smoked Salmon in Scrambled Eggs

Lunch: Butternut Squash Carrot Soup

Dinner: Bulgur Kale Pesto Salad

Snack: Ginger-Cinnamon Mixed Nuts

Day 9

Breakfast: Spinach and Potatoes with Smoked Salmon

Lunch: Kale Quinoa Shrimp Bowl

Dinner: Salmon Roast with Romaine and Potatoes

Snack: Ginger Date Almond Bars

Day 10

Breakfast: Eggs in a Mushroom and Bacon

Lunch: Egg Bowl and Veggies

Dinner: Bean Bolognese

Snack: Coffee Cacao Protein Bars

Day 11

Breakfast: Bacon Avocado Burger

Lunch: Turkey Taco Bowls

Dinner: Peppers Stuffed with Sweet Potato

and Turkey

Snack: Turmeric Gummies

Day 12

Breakfast: Spinach Fry Up & Tomato Mushroom

Lunch: Bulgur Kale Pesto Salad

Dinner: Turkey Meatballs

Snack: Ginger-Cinnamon Mixed Nuts

Day 13

Breakfast: Chocolate Milkshake

Lunch: Turkish Scrambled Eggs

Dinner: Chicken Chili and White Beans

Snack: Ginger Date Almond Bars

Day 14

Breakfast: Almond Sweet Cherry Chia Pudding

Lunch: Swiss Chard and Red Lentil Curried Soup

Dinner: Cauliflower Rice and Salmon Bowl

Snack: Coffee Cacao Protein Bars

Day 15

Breakfast: Shakshuka

Lunch: Orange Cardamom Quinoa with Carrots

Dinner: Harissa and Chicken Tenders

Snack: Turmeric Gummies

Day 17

Breakfast: Amaranth Porridge with Pears

Lunch: Tomato Stew with Chickpea and Kale

Dinner: Baked Cauliflower Buffalo

Snack: Turmeric Gummies

Day 19

Breakfast: Apple Turkey Hash

Lunch: Salmon with Veggies Sheet Pan

Dinner:

Lentil Soup with Lemons

Snack: Ginger-Cinnamon Mixed Nuts

Day 21

Breakfast: Chia Energy Bars with Chocolate

Lunch: Garlic Tomato Basil Chicken

Dinner: Asian Garlic Noodles

Snack: Turmeric Gummies

Day 16

Breakfast: Anti-Inflammatory Salad

Lunch: Quinoa Turmeric Power Bowl

Dinner: Chinese Chicken Salad

Snack: Ginger Date Almond Bars

Day 18

Breakfast: Sweet Potato Breakfast Bowl

Lunch: Anti-Inflammatory Beef Meatballs

Dinner: Kale and Sweet Potato Tostadas

Snack: Coffee Cacao Protein Bars

Day 20

Breakfast: Oats with Almonds and Blueberries

Lunch: Shrimp Fajitas

Dinner: Mediterranean One Pan Cod

Snack: Ginger Date Almond Bars

Day 22

Breakfast: Baked Rice Porridge with Maple and Fruit

Lunch: Shrimp Garlic Zoodles

Dinner: Cauliflower Grits and Shrimp

Snack: Ginger Date Almond Bars

Day 23

Breakfast: Banana Chia Pudding

Dinner: Stir-Fried Snap Pea and Chicken

Snack: Turmeric Gummies

Day 24

Lunch: Green Curry

Breakfast: Baked Eggs with Herbs

Lunch: Turkey Chili with Avocado

Dinner: Turkey Chili with Avocado

Snack: Coffee Cacao Protein Bars

Day 25

Breakfast: Banana Bread Pecan Overnight Oats

Lunch: Grecian-Style Turkey Burgers

with Tzatziki

Dinner: Chicken with Lemon and Asparagus

Snack: Ginger-Cinnamon Mixed Nuts

Day 26

Breakfast: Cinnamon Granola with Fruits

Lunch: Bean Bolognese

Dinner: Bean Bolognese

Snack: Turmeric Gummies

Day 27

Breakfast: Yogurt Parfait with Chia Seeds

and Raspberries

Lunch: Peppers Stuffed with Sweet Potato and Turkey

Dinner: Harissa and Chicken Tenders

Snack: Ginger Date Almond Bars

Day 28

Breakfast: Avocado Toast with Egg

Lunch: Roasted Sweet Potatoes with Avocado Dip

Dinner: Kale and Sweet Potato Tostadas

Snack: Turmeric Gummies

Day 29

Breakfast: Winter Morning Breakfast Bowl

Lunch: Chicken Chili and White Beans

Dinner: Lentil Soup with Lemons

Snack: Coffee Cacao Protein Bars

Day 30

Breakfast: Broccoli and Quinoa Breakfast Patties

Lunch: Mediterranean One Pan Cod

Dinner: Asian Garlic Noodles

Snack: Ginger-Cinnamon Mixed Nuts

Conclusion

Arguably, the most healthful dietary regimen revolves around a plant-centric approach. Vegetarians and vegans often contend with unfounded stereotypes of frailty or poor health, particularly from carnivores and aficionados of budget-friendly fare. These stereotypes represent mere misconceptions, unfounded assumptions perpetuated by those unfamiliar with vegetarianism or plant-based cuisine. Contrary to these myths, the majority of vegetables and other natural components prevalent in the diet of vegetarians or vegans are notably rich in nutrients while being low in calories. Beyond exceptional nutritional value, anti-inflammatory diets demonstrate positive health outcomes, including reduced susceptibility to cancer, heart disease, and type 2 diabetes.

The second Adventist Health Study, reflecting compelling evidence, highlights that vegetarians and vegans exhibit a median weight loss of 35 pounds in comparison to their meat-consuming counterparts. It is imperative to discern reality from the unfounded claims surrounding the health benefits derived from plant-derived sustenance. Undoubtedly, there are substantial advantages associated with the consumption of food sourced directly from the earth.

Made in United States
Troutdale, OR
04/08/2024